Frontline Cardiology

An off-the-fence guide for those who need
a definitive answer to "What do I do next?"

Nick Fisher MBBS, MRCP, MD

Consultant Interventional Cardiologist,
North Hampshire Hospital, Basingstoke,
Hampshire, UK

Surgeon Commander, Royal Navy, UK

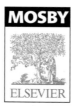

MOSBY

ELSEVIER

MOSBY
ELSEVIER

First published 2006

ISBN-10: 0-7234-3425-5
ISBN-13: 978-0-7234-3425-2

British Library Cataloguing in Publication Data
A catalogue record for this book is available from the British Library

Library of Congress Cataloging in Publication Data
A catalogue record for this book is available from the Library of Congress

Notice
Knowledge and best practice in this field are constantly changing. As new research and experience broaden our knowledge, changes in practice, treatment and drug therapy may become necessary or appropriate. Readers are advised to check the most current information provided (i) on procedures featured or (ii) by the manufacturer of each product to be administered, to verify the recommended dose or formula, the method and duration of administration, and contraindications. It is the responsibility of the practitioner, relying on their own experience and knowledge of the patient, to make diagnoses, to determine dosages and the best treatment for each individual patient, and to take all appropriate safety precautions. To the fullest extent of the law, neither the publisher nor the author assumes any liability for any injury and/or damage.

The views expressed in this publication are those of the author(s) and not necessarily those of the publisher or the sponsors.

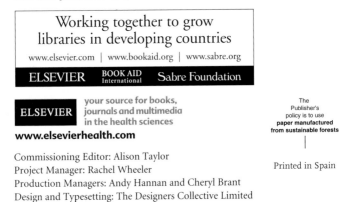

Working together to grow
libraries in developing countries

www.elsevier.com | www.bookaid.org | www.sabre.org

ELSEVIER   BOOK AID International   Sabre Foundation

ELSEVIER   your source for books, journals and multimedia in the health sciences

www.elsevierhealth.com

The Publisher's policy is to use **paper manufactured from sustainable forests**

Commissioning Editor: Alison Taylor
Project Manager: Rachel Wheeler
Production Managers: Andy Hannan and Cheryl Brant
Design and Typesetting: The Designers Collective Limited

Printed in Spain

Cover image: Zephyr/Science Photo Library

Dedication

I would like to dedicate this book to my wife and children and to my parents, who have supported me throughout my career.

Additional contributors

Emma Birks Cardiology SPR, Royal Brompton Hospital, London, UK

Simon Davies Consultant Cardiologist, Royal Brompton Hospital, London, UK

Jeff Davison Senior Technician, Royal Brompton Hospital, London, UK

Malcolm Finlay Cardiology SHO, Royal Brompton Hospital, London, UK

Mike Gatzoulis Professor, Grown Up Congenital Heart Disease, Royal Brompton Hospital, London, UK

Derek Gibson Consultant Cardiologist, Royal Brompton Hospital, London, UK

Bilal Iqbal Cardiology SHO, Royal Brompton Hospital, London, UK

Janet Lock Senior Pharmacist, North Hampshire Hospital, Basingstoke, Hampshire, UK

Mike Mullen Consultant, Grown Up Congenital Heart Disease, Royal Brompton Hospital, London, UK

Tammy Pegg Cardiology SPR, North Hampshire Hospital, Basingstoke, UK

John Pepper Professor, Cardiothoracic Surgery, Royal Brompton Hospital, London, UK

Susanna Price Cardiology SPR, Royal Brompton Hospital, London, UK

Hayley Pryse-Hawkins Heart Failure Nurse, Royal Brompton Hospital, London, UK

Richard Sutton Consultant Cardiologist, Royal Brompton Hospital, London, UK

Contents

Preface

This is not a textbook and it would serve you poorly if used as such. It is a homunculus of cardiology knowledge, based on our experiences, with the sole aim of helping you to make a decision when faced with the daily challenges of cardiology.

We live in an age where access to the latest trial data is immediate. For many clinicians, lack of knowledge is not the problem; instead it is inadequate experience that holds them back from making a decision based on that knowledge. I call this 'evidence-based paralysis'. Sometimes you don't want to know what a group of experts decided in the latest 'aren't we great trial'; you simply want to know what to do next.

Obviously there is no substitute for experience, but to help you along the way our aim is to help you get off the fence and to indicate what we have done in similar situations. We are not going to teach you how to do an angioplasty or put in a pacemaker. We will tell you when a patient should have one, what the problems may be and how you should deal with them. You will not find phrases like 'consider an anti-arrhythmic', because I assume that if you were doing so you have turned to this book!

Also, it is our sincere intention to offer evidence-based advice, but we have actively avoided death by trial data. Some may disagree with our statements or algorithms and that is obviously the danger of the off-the-fence approach; clearly, because you can't be in everyone's garden at the same time, someone has to be unhappy. That's life and we don't claim to be experts. But remember that one definition of an expert is someone who has made all the mistakes that there are to be made in a very small field.

Finally, if you disagree with the content of this book, feel you could have done it better or would like something added and have finished telling everyone else the fact (a genetic certainty with most cardiologists), please let me know so we can continue to improve the book in the spirit that it was written.

Nick Fisher MBBS, MRCP, MD
Consultant Interventional Cardiologist
Surgeon Commander, Royal Navy

Acute coronary syndromes

chapter
1

Nick Fisher
Tammy Pegg
Simon Davies

INTRODUCTION

This is a basic guide for managing acute coronary syndromes (ACS) and has been developed using guidelines from the European Society of Cardiology and the National Institute for Health and Clinical Excellence. We set out how to diagnose, risk stratify and manage ACS with the least fuss possible.

DEFINITION

ACS have been redefined many times and are often confusing. For the time being you should consider ACS as a spectrum of clinical conditions presenting as chest pain, which include unstable angina at one end and ST elevation myocardial infarction (STEMI) at the other.

DIAGNOSIS

Please don't use the troponin level alone to diagnose ACS (see **Table 1**), and remember that having chest pain is central to making the diagnosis. Other features, such as electrocardiogram (ECG) changes and troponin levels, can be normal (**Table 2**).

"Have I had a heart attack doctor?"

If making an exact diagnosis of myocardial infarction is important to the patient (for example for insurance purposes, driving or

Table 1. Pitfalls of relying on troponin level tests

- Absence of troponin does not exclude coronary heart disease
- Other conditions may cause elevated troponin levels, for example:
  - Pneumonia
  - Pulmonary embolus
  - Myopericarditis
  - Myocardial contusions
  - Renal failure
  - Arrhythmia, including atrial fibrillation

Table 2. Diagnostic features of acute coronary syndromes

	Troponin T/I	ECG
Unstable angina*	< 0.05	• ST↓ • Transient ST↑ • T waves↓ • Normal
Non-STEMI	> 0.05	• ST↓ • Transient ST↑ • T waves↓ • Normal
STEMI	> 0.05	• Persistent ST↑

*Unstable angina without ECG changes must be qualified by a previous history of coronary artery

work) you should be pragmatic. A practical cut-off for 'heart attack' is:

- Troponin T > 1.0 ng/ml or
- Troponin I > 0.5 ng/ml.

These levels have been demonstrated to have similar mortality and left ventricular dysfunction as the previous World Health Organisation classification of myocardial infarction (creatinine kinase > 400 iu/l).

HOW TO RISK STRATIFY THE PATIENT

Risk stratification is an important tool to help identify patients at risk of further chest pain or complications. Various scores have been shown to identify high-risk patients who benefit from early aggressive therapy and revascularisation. The Global Registry of Acute Coronary Events (GRACE registry) and Thrombolysis in Myocardial Infarction (TIMI) risk scores have been demonstrated to predict outcome in ACS.

The easiest to use is the TIMI score (**Table 3**). Each point scores one mark; add up the total for each patient for an approximate major adverse event rate at six months (see **Table 4**).

PATHOPHYSIOLOGY

In most cases, ACS is caused by the rupture of an unstable atheromatous plaque. Therefore, the principles of treatment for STEMI and unstable angina are broadly the same:

- Prevention or dissolution of acute thrombus
- Prevention of secondary complications of myocardial damage
- Plaque stabilisation.

Table 3. The TIMI risk score

Patients score one point for each of the following*:
- Age > 65 years
- More than three risk factors for ACS:
  - Smoking
  - Diabetes
  - Raised blood pressure
  - Angina
- Documented coronary stenosis > 50%
- ST deviation
- More than two anginal events in 24 hours
- Prior aspirin use
- Increased cardiac enzymes

*Maximum score = 7

Table 4. Using the TIMI risk score to predict major event rate at six months

TIMI risk score	% Death/myocardial infarction	% Death/myocardial infarction/ revascularisation
0/1	3	5
2	3	8
3	5	13
4	7	20
5	12	26
6/7	19	41

Despite their common cause, however, treatment is classically very different. We have therefore dealt with acute STEMI in Chapter 4 (note that this situation is likely to change in the future).

FIRST-LINE TREATMENT
Oxygen
You won't find any drug reps pushing oxygen, but it's still around, working as well as ever, and anaesthetists swear by it! Don't get l/min confused with %. Ask for the maximum.

Diamorphine 2.5–5 mg i.v. titrated slowly with 10 mg metoclopramide i.v.
Giving adequate analgesia makes both the patient and the doctor feel more comfortable. It removes the adrenaline response to acute illness, thereby reducing the patient's pulse rate and blood pressure. This:
- Prevents adrenaline-driven arrhythmias
- Maximises diastolic coronary perfusion
- Reduces afterload on the heart.

Aspirin 300 mg orally, followed by 75 mg daily
This is often given by the GP or by paramedics, but it is important that you ensure it has been administered.

Nitrates

Glyceryl trinitrate (GTN) i.v. is usually available as a 50 ml infusion. Start it at an infusion rate of 0.6 ml/h and titrate to a maximum of 10 ml/h. Aim to keep systolic blood pressure > 100 mmHg.

Beta blockers

These can be given intravenously in the accident and emergency department, and are particularly helpful for hypertensive and tachycardic patients who have not settled with intravenous diamorphine.

Give 1–5 mg i.v. metoprolol (short acting) slowly over 3 minutes, titrated to pulse and blood pressure. Be wary of atrioventricular (AV) block, asthma and acute left ventricular failure.

Enoxaparin 1 mg/kg bd or dalteparin bd

Use a weight-adjusted dose (see charts). Low molecular weight heparin (LMWH) is superior to unfractionated (UF) heparin. Although studies have shown that percutaneous transluminal coronary angioplasty can also be performed safely with LMWH, there is some concern that we cannot monitor the activated partial thromboplastin time (APTT) or actual clotting time (ACT). Most clinicians have therefore adapted the approach of stabilising patients on LMWH, but omitting it on the morning of the procedure. This is replaced with i.v. UF heparin during angioplasty, if necessary, and allows accurate titration to ACT.

SECOND-LINE TREATMENT

You should now know the exact diagnosis and understand whether the patient is at low, intermediate or high risk of future adverse cardiac events. You should make appropriate plans for long-term management and revascularisation.

If the patient is a candidate for revascularisation they should receive the following drugs.

Clopidogrel

- Give clopidogrel 300 mg immediately
- Load with clopidogrel 600 mg if you anticipate rapid transfer for cardiac angiography (< 6 hours)
- Continue with clopidogrel 75 mg od until after the cardiac angiogram (**Table 5**).

Table 5. Giving clopidogrel as second-line treatment	
Outcome of cardiac angiogram treatment	**Duration of clopidogrel**
Medical treatment	1 year unless caution applies
Coronary artery bypass graft	Discontinue
Stent	Variable depending on stent

Glycoprotein IIb/IIIa inhibitors

Patients who show most benefit from glycoprotein IIb/IIIa inhibitors (and who should therefore be started on these drugs) are those with:

- Diabetes
- Dynamic ST segment changes
- Possible delay to their percutaneous coronary intervention (PCI) (i.e. over the weekend)
- Recurrent pain despite optimal treatment.

Dosages are as follows:

- Abciximab: 250 mcg/kg i.v. bolus then 125 ng/kg/min for up to 24 hours
- Tirofiban: 0.4 mcg/kg i.v. bolus then 0.1 mcg/kg infusion for up to 48 hours. (If started in the cardiac catheterisation lab 10 mcg/kg bolus with a 0.15 mcg/kg/min infusion 12–24 h)
- Eptifibatide: 180 mcg/kg bolus followed by continuous infusion of 2 mcg/kg/min for 48 hours.

Tables 6 and 7 list the contraindications and what to do if bleeding complications occur.

Table 6. Contraindications to glycoprotein IIb/IIIa inhibitors

In the last 2 months	In last 2 years	Lifetime history
• Active bleeding • Major surgery • Intracranial/spinal surgery	• Stroke	• Intracranial neoplasm • AV malformation/aneurysm • Diabetic retinopathy • Severe hypertension • Thrombocytopenia

Table 7. Managing bleeding complications

How to avoid them:
- Check the platelet count daily and stop the infusion if < 100 x 10^9/l

What to do:
- Stop the glycoprotein IIb/IIIa inhibitor
- Check the platelet count:
  - If the bleed is significant or continuous you can give platelets, but this won't make any difference with tirofiban or eptifibatide
- Cross match the patient for blood and replace what is lost

Don't panic, most patients will stop bleeding:
- If a puncture site haematoma is not controlled with a Femstop, speak with the vascular surgeons
- If the patient has a gastrointestinal haemorrhage speak with the gastroenterologists

Other treatments
Proton pump inhibitors
We have adopted a policy of using routine, short-term, proton pump inhibitors to cover stress ulceration in patients with ACS, as follows:

- Omeprazole 20 mg od continued for one month after discharge.

Beta blockers
Use:

- Atenolol 50 mg for men
- Atenolol 25 mg for small women.

Take care in patients with:

- Asthma
- AV block
- Left ventricular failure.

If in any doubt use metoprolol 12.5 mg tds titrated up accordingly. If this is well tolerated, switch to atenolol because compliance is better with once-daily treatment.

Statins
The principle of statin treatment is to start high and reassess. They are indicated for all patients with ACS, even those with a normal baseline cholesterol. Our protocol is as follows:

- Give 40 mg of simvastatin or equivalent
- Reassess cholesterol at three months
- Aim for a total cholesterol of < 4.5 mmol/l and a low-density lipoprotein cholesterol of < 2.5 mmol/l.

In suitable patients we may start with a very high dose of atorvastatin (80 mg), then convert to a standard regime after three months.

Angiotensin converting enzyme inhibitors
Angiotensin converting enzyme (ACE) inhibitors received much positive publicity for use in patients with myocardial infarction

complicated by left ventricular failure. Further research has extended their role to patients with ACS.

They are thought to act on endothelium. They stabilise plaque disease as well as being effective remodelling agents and antihypertensives.

Dosages are as follows:
- Perindopril 2 mg, 4 mg, 8 mg
- Ramipril 1.25 mg, 2.5 mg, 5 mg, 10 mg.

Patients with diabetes

There were no data for ACS in the DIGAMI study,[1] except for patients with acute myocardial infarction. Sensibly it would seem wise to extend the protocol to include non-STEMI.

For patients with new or established diabetes or with a glucose level > 11.0 mmol/l on admission we prescribe:
- 50 units of Actrapid in 50 ml of 0.9% NaCl adjusted to a sliding scale
- 5% dextrose 30 ml/h.

Aim for a target blood glucose of 5.0–10.0 mmol/l.

Dosages of insulin are given in **Table 8**. If a patient needs a high dose of i.v. insulin and you need to convert them to subcutaneous insulin before the diabetes team has reviewed the patient, a reasonable approach is:
- Mixtard 30/70 0.5 units/kg in two divided doses (2/3 given in the morning, 1/3 given with the evening meal).

THIRD-LINE TREATMENT
Anti-anginal agents

Your back should be against the pharmacological wall by this stage. Adding an anti-anginal beyond a beta blocker should mean that you are considering intervention and looking for interim stabilisation, or that the patient is not suitable for intervention.

Table 8. Administering intravenous insulin	
Blood glucose (mmol/l)	**Insulin (ml/h)**
> 20.0	4.0
15.1–20.0	3.0
10.1–15.0	2.0
5.0–10.0	1.0
< 5.0	0.5
< 3.0	Stop temporarily

Nitrates

Maintaining patients long term on an i.v. infusion is not recommended. If further nitrate is needed, you should switch to an oral preparation as soon as the patient can tolerate this, as follows:

- Isosorbide mononitrate 10 mg, 20 mg, 30 mg bd.

Remember to ensure a nitrate-free period to avoid tolerance, so prescribe in the morning and at lunch.

Potassium channel activators

These are normally well tolerated and have few interactions with other anti-anginal medications. We use:

- Nicorandil 10 mg
- Titration to 30 mg bd.

Calcium channel antagonists

Dosages are as follows:

- Diltiazem 120 mg, 180 mg, 240 mg XL
  - Use diltiazem if the heart rate is not too slow because it blocks the AV node
- Amlodipine 5–10 mg
  - Use if the heart rate is too slow or if the patient is on a beta blocker
  - Amlodipine can cause non-cardiac peripheral oedema (try felodipine).

REVASCULARISATION

With the support of glycoprotein IIb/IIIa antagonists and coronary stents, early intervention is now recommended.

Inpatient intervention should be your first option in patients with all forms of ACS, especially those with:

- Recurrent angina (at rest or with minimal effort)
- Increased enzyme levels
- New ST depression or left bundle branch block
- New signs of left ventricular failure, decreased ejection fraction or low blood pressure
- Previous percutaneous transluminal coronary intervention.

This also applies to anyone else with a strongly positive exercise ECG or nuclear perfusion scan. Important points to remember are listed in **Table 9.**

Table 9. Revascularisation: points to remember

- Coronary intervention is not a risk-free procedure. You should not regard moving a patient to the cardiac catheterisation lab as a thankful knee-jerk next step that gets a patient off your hands (as some clinicians regard moving patients to the intensive care unit!)

- Narrowed coronary arteries are not the only cause of angina. Consider other factors such as:
  - Anaemia
  - High-output states related to arrhythmias or thyrotoxicosis
  - Severe aortic stenosis

- Kidneys don't 'like' contrast media used in cardiac catheterisation labs. Patients with poor renal function can be pushed into renal failure

- Don't send your 92-year-old female patient with an uncomplicated myocardial infarction, anaemia, a haemoglobin of 8.2 g/l, a creatinine of 332 µmol/l and a recent perforated duodenal ulcer straight to the cardiac catheterisation lab

Coronary angiography

Nick Fisher
Simon Davies

INTRODUCTION

Coronary angiography is the most definitive investigation for assessing coronary artery patency. Other techniques (such as contrast echocardiography) may be able to determine myocardial perfusion more accurately, but unless perfusion is normal you will still need to determine the severity and extent of coronary artery disease before starting management.

A modern invasive strategy using the medications outlined in Chapter 1 reduces death, myocardial infarction, symptoms and readmission.

BEFORE SENDING THE PATIENT TO THE CARDIAC CATHETERISATION LAB

The steps to follow are described below.

Consent

The risk of complications following angiography and angioplasty are listed in **Table 10**.

Document

Biochemistry

Document the results of the following biochemistry tests:

- International normalised ratio (INR)
- Haemoglobin
- Platelets

Table 10. Risk of complications (%)

	Angiography	Angioplasty
Pain/bruising	10.0	20.0
Haematoma	2.0	5.0
Arterial damage	1.0	1.0
Stroke	0.5	0.5
Myocardial infarction	0.5	1.0
Death	0.1	0.5

- Urea
- Creatinine.

Renal dysfunction

If creatinine is > 150 µmol/l, give N-acetylcysteine (600 mg before the procedure and 600 mg bd in the 24 hours following the procedure). If the patient is likely to have a long wait, put up i.v. fluids.

Previous contrast reaction

Ask the patient whether they have ever had a reaction to contrast agents. If they have, document it in detail.

Metformin

Discontinue metformin on the day of the angiography. Do not restart until 48 hours later and after urea and electrolytes show normal renal function. If the pre-angiography level was abnormal, do not restart metformin.

Grafts

If the patient has had a previous graft, find out where and obtain the operation notes. *Don't let a patient go to the lab without operation notes unless the operator has been informed.* The reason for this paranoia is that serious damage has been caused by operators fishing around for grafts that don't exist, or that are in different places than initially thought.

Previous angiography
Determine:
- What approach was used
- What it showed
- Whether grafts were patent
- Whether an Angioseal device was used (you cannot use the same approach for three months after an Angioseal has been used).

Peripheral vascular disease
Check the patient's peripheral pulses and history of claudication, and find out whether they have had vascular surgery, especially on the aorta and femoral arteries. Check for abdominal aortic aneurysms.

THINK: should the patient have a brachial/radial approach?

Prescribe
Prescribe the following drugs:
- Clopidogrel (if the patient is not on it already)
  - 300 mg stat if angioplasty is likely
  - 600 mg if going to the lab that day
- Prophylactic antibiotics if the patient has a metallic valve.

WHEN THE PATIENT RETURNS TO THE WARD
Close femoral puncture sites
The steps to follow are:
- Apply pressure
- Deploy a Femstop
- Deploy a Starclose/Angioseal/Perclose.

These are described below.

Pressure

As always, you can make things easy for yourself by taking time to prepare, as follows:
- Lower the bed or stand on a stool so that you can press with straight arms
- Get some gauze
- Make sure someone else is around in case you get into trouble
- Have atropine handy in case the patient has a vagal attack.
- Do you know that the ACT is less than 150 seconds and that the systolic blood pressure is lower than 150 mmHg?
- A little lignocaine is nice if the sheath has been in for some time.

During the procedure:
- Place the fingertips of your non-dominant hand over the puncture site
- Angle inwards slightly allowing for the fact that the femoral artery heads towards the midline
- Remove the sheath with one confident pull, pressing with your other hand as it leaves the artery to prevent bleeding
- Support your non-dominant hand by placing the tips of your other hand on it
- Keep your arms straight and press for 10 minutes
- You should prevent bleeding, but there should still be a faint popliteal pulse because you are not trying to produce an ischaemic limb, and you need a bit of blood flow to help clotting at the puncture site.

The patient should lie flat for at least 1 hour. They may get up after 3–6 hours, depending on the size of the sheath. (Make yourself aware of the ward's arterial sheath policy.)

Femstop

Find a nurse who knows how to deploy a Femstop. The key points to remember are:

- The device should be positioned so that you can see the puncture site
- The device should not stop you from palpating the peripheral pulses
- A staff member should be allocated to oversee the gradual deflation of the Femstop.

The patient should lie flat for at least 4 hours after the device is removed.

There is a graph on the back of the Femstop packet to help with the deflation procedure. In a nutshell:

- Inflate the cuff until 20 mmHg above systolic
- Confirm there is no bleeding
- Ease off the pressure until you can feel a pedal pulse
- Leave it for 15 minutes
- Drop 20 mmHg below systolic for 2 minutes and then another 20 mmHg for another 2 minutes
- Leave for 20 minutes at about 30 mmHg before removing the Femstop.

Starclose/Angioseal/Perclose

This will have been deployed at the time of the procedure. The operator should have documented the presence of peripheral pulses at deployment. Sometimes they can ooze and gentle proximal pressure is normally all that is needed.

In theory the patient can walk straight away but, if possible, you should advise them to lie flat for at least 2 hours.

Manage haematomas

Patients have died after coronary angiography because of neglected haematomas. A certain amount of bruising around a femoral puncture site is acceptable, as is a small haematoma.

Larger haematomas can be dissipated by firm pressure for 5–10 minutes. What you must not miss is a pulsatile swelling, especially with a bruit that may represent a false aneurysm. If in doubt, ask for an ultrasound.

Radiologists will treat false aneurysms in one of two ways:
- By applying direct pressure with their probe to ensure that they have stopped flow in the aneurysm
- By injecting with thrombin, which causes the false lumen to clot almost immediately.

However, if the neck of the aneurysm is too large then surgical closure by the vascular surgeons will be necessary.

Rehydrate the patient
Make sure that patients (who may have been 'nil by mouth' for some time) have access to water and are encouraged to drink. This is especially important for patients with poor renal function because contrast media can cause further deterioration.

Have a low threshold for giving i.v. fluids if the patient is unlikely or unable to drink. Be aware of poor left ventricular function when determining the rate and the type of fluid.

Read the notes
Remember that angiography is a diagnostic not therapeutic procedure. Check whether there were any complications during the procedure and whether further treatment recommendations have been made in the lab, for example a request for:
- A surgical opinion
- Thallium or magnetic resonance imaging (MRI) scans
- Medication change(s).

chapter 3

Angioplasty

Nick Fisher
Simon Davies

INTRODUCTION

The ideal situation for angioplasty is single vessel disease with a focal stenosis, but the safety and efficacy of direct stenting of lesions with the cover of glycoprotein IIb/IIIa inhibitors has now blurred the boundaries for surgery.

However, severe triple vessel disease and left main disease is still more frequently referred for surgery because losing a significant vessel during a PCI would not be adequately compensated for by the collaterals from the other diseased arteries. In certain cases, where the risk of immediate surgery is considered unacceptable, a PCI may be attempted on the culprit lesion as a palliative procedure.

The angiogram is typically reported as a stick diagram in the notes, indicating the vessel affected, extent of stenosis and TIMI flow (**Figure 1**). Sites of stenoses are marked and stent width, length and make will be recorded.

TIMI flow is graded as follows:
- Grade 0 = no flow
- Grade 1 = minimal flow with no distal arterial perfusion
- Grade 2 = entire vessel perfused, but sluggish flow compared with normal vessels
- Grade 3 = normal.

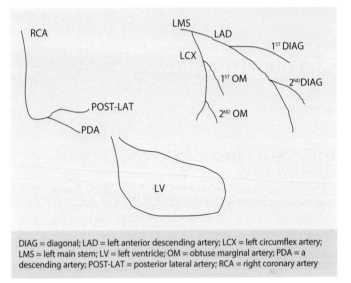

DIAG = diagonal; LAD = left anterior descending artery; LCX = left circumflex artery; LMS = left main stem; LV = left ventricle; OM = obtuse marginal artery; PDA = a descending artery; POST-LAT = posterior lateral artery; RCA = right coronary artery

Figure 1.
Standard stick diagram of coronary arteries commonly drawn by cardiologists along with indication of left ventricular dimension and function.

STENTS

Plain old balloon angioplasty resulted in improved symptoms compared with medical treatment, but because of early failure (often due to re-stenosis in about 35% of cases) surgery was better in short- and medium-term follow-ups.

Stents, however, have a higher success rate. They have lower rates of:

- Re-stenosis (15%)
- Target lesion revascularisation
- Clinical events at 1 year.

Coated stents

The Cypher Sirolimus stent has a naturally occurring macrocyclic lactone, which is used as an immunosuppressive and anti-proliferative agent. Stents coated with this lactone have attracted the most recent attention because they significantly reduce the incidence of in-stent restenosis.

When these stents are used there is a greater likelihood that reduced endothelial growth will leave the stent metalwork exposed for longer. Therefore, clopidogrel should be continued for at least 6 months after implantation of a drug-eluting stent, and 1 month for a bare metal stent.

ROTATIONAL ATHERECTOMY (ROTABLATOR)

This gadget consists of an elliptical burr coated with diamond microparticles welded to a metal drive shaft that track along a guide wire. The shaft is rotated by an air turbine at speeds of up to 200,000 rpm. It is suitable for short, heavily calcified lesions that would not expand with a conventional PCI. The residual lumen is normally about 80% of the reference and is further dilated with a PCI at the end of the procedure.

COMPLICATIONS OF PERCUTANEOUS CORONARY INTERVENTIONS

Routine use of stents and glycoprotein IIb/IIIa inhibitors has made PCIs a safe and effective way of treating ACS.

Acute occlusion

Acute occlusion of the target vessel can occur in up to 8% of patients. Most cases occur within 24 hours and are usually the result of dissection. In 75% of patients this becomes apparent on the table, and if it is not extensive it may be treated by placing another (distal) stent.

Thrombosis

With the use of aspirin and clopidogrel, thrombosis now occurs in less than 2% of patients.

Chronic occlusion

Chronic occlusion (i.e. re-stenosis) occurs mainly in the first four months, and if not present by six months it is unlikely to occur.

Small vessels have a higher incidence of re-stenosis, especially in patients with diabetes.

CLOPIDOGREL

All patients undergoing angioplasty and not already receiving clopidogrel should be given a 300 mg loading dose if they are going to the lab the next day, or 600 mg if going the same day.

Points to consider include:
- For uncoated, bare metal stents clopidogrel should be continued for at least 1 month
- For the currently available drug-eluting stents clopidogrel should be continued for at least 6 months, and then reviewed according to current guidelines (it may need to be given indefinitely). This reflects the significant risk of in-stent thrombosis in the absence of aspirin and clopidogrel due to exposed stent struts
- Studies of ACS recommend that patients take clopidogrel for 12 months. Therefore, many centres prescribe it for all patients for this time regardless of stent insertion or type, particularly when the intervention took place in the setting of an ACS
- Some patients with significant diffuse disease who suffer repeated ACS should receive lifelong clopidogrel
- Patients should not receive aspirin, clopidogrel and warfarin together. Patients who are receiving warfarin for atrial fibrillation should stop the warfarin in the week before angioplasty and start aspirin and clopidogrel. The clopidogrel timings should remain unchanged
- If the patient is receiving warfarin for a metal valve or significant embolic risk, warfarin should be continued and aspirin omitted. The clopidogrel timings should remain unchanged.

Myocardial infarction

Nick Fisher
Tammy Pegg
Simon Davies

INTRODUCTION

This chapter deals specifically with diagnosing and managing acute myocardial infarction, which includes:

- STEMI
- True posterior myocardial infarction
- New left bundle branch block.

DIAGNOSIS

Patients should have pain consistent with an infarct and significant ECG changes (**Table 11**). Repeat serial ECGs (at least every 10 minutes, depending on suspicion).

Table 11. ECG changes compatible with acute myocardial infarction

- 1 mm ST elevation in two or more contiguous limb leads (pain within 12 hours)

- 2 mm ST elevation in two or more contiguous chest leads (pain within 12 hours)

- New or presumed new left bundle branch block (pain within 6 hours)

- ST depression in V1–4, with dominant R wave in V1 compatible with posterior myocardial infarction (pain within 6 hours)

NB. Turn the ECG upside down and face down. Now hold it up to the light. A posterior myocardial infarction will look like an anterior STEMI.

Remember:

- Subtle ST elevation can look like high take-off
- But high take-off is **NOT** dynamic, i.e. it does not increase or change with subsequent ECGs
- Echocardiography can often show a regional wall abnormality, and of course a coronary artery angiogram can show the occlusion
- ST elevation without chest pain **DOES NOT** require thrombolysis
- Left ventricular aneurysm tends to produce fixed ST elevation in the presence of Q waves in anterior chest leads. This can be confused with new ST elevation
- Pan- or saddle-shaped ST elevation could be pericarditis
- Ask for help.

FIRST-LINE TREATMENT

Some of the information we have given here is the same as the advice given for ACS in Chapter 1. We feel the repetition is worthwhile to save you turning between the two chapters, and there are also some important differences.

Oxygen

You won't find any drug reps pushing oxygen, but it's still around, working as well as ever, and anaesthetists swear by it! Don't get l/min confused with %. Ask for the maximum.

Diamorphine 2.5–5 mg i.v. titrated slowly with 10 mg metoclopramide i.v.

Giving adequate analgesia makes both the patient and the doctor feel more comfortable. It removes the adrenaline response to acute illness, thereby reducing the patient's pulse rate and blood pressure. This:

- Prevents adrenaline-driven arrhythmias
- Maximises diastolic coronary perfusion
- Reduces afterload on the heart.

Aspirin 300 mg orally, followed by 75 mg daily

This is often given by the GP or by paramedics, but it is important that you ensure it has been administered.

Clopidogrel 300 mg stat

This drug should be given to patients with the aspirin.

Nitrates

GTN i.v. is usually available as a 50 ml infusion. Start it at an infusion rate of 0.6 ml/h and titrate to a maximum of 10 ml/h. Aim to keep systolic blood pressure > 100 mmHg.

Beta blockers

These can be given intravenously in the accident and emergency department, and are particularly helpful for hypertensive and tachycardic patients who have not settled with intravenous diamorphine.

Give 1–5 mg i.v. metoprolol (short acting) slowly over 3 minutes, titrated to pulse and blood pressure. Be wary of AV block, asthma and acute left ventricular failure.

REVASCULARISATION WITH PRIMARY ANGIOPLASTY

Primary angioplasty is now preferable to thrombolysis (**Table 12**). This procedure is becoming more common, but in many centres it

---

Table 12. Benefits of PCI over thrombolysis

- Increased target vessel patency
- Provides the ultimate diagnostic test for acute myocardial infarction and avoids inappropriate treatment
- Almost non-existent incidence of intracranial haemorrhage
- Reduced incidence of re-infarction

is available only during the working day. In these cases, thrombolysis followed by angiography the following day often occurs (facilitated angioplasty). This may turn out to be a perfectly acceptable long-term approach.

You should seek out-of-hours primary angioplasty for patients with:
- Cardiogenic shock
- Contraindications to thrombolysis
- Large anterior myocardial infarcts.

Remember:
- Transfer to the cardiac catheterisation lab is not the same as transfer to the intensive care unit
- The potential benefits should outweigh the risks
- The patient will need to lie flat for over an hour
- The patient's airway must be secure before transfer and their breathing should be stable
- The patient will need to be compliant with treatment
- You should consider an acute myocardial infarction within the whole clinical context.

Drugs

Load the patient with:
- Aspirin 300 mg (ventilated patients will need a nasogastric tube)
- Clopidogrel 600 mg (ventilated patients will need a nasogastric tube).

Start the patient on a glycoprotein IIb/IIIa inhibitor (tirofiban: see Chapter 1 for doses).

Don't forget:
- Use a large Venflon
- Do routine blood tests, including 'group and save'
- Gain the patient's consent.

REVASCULARISATION WITH THROMBOLYSIS

If primary angioplasty is not available, then the old favourite is still very effective. Most of us now use a single bolus of tenecteplase 30–50 mg (according to body weight) i.v. over 10 seconds. This is easy to draw up and administer. Pre-treat with 5000 units of heparin. Patients must also receive a treatment dose of enoxaparin (1 mg/kg bd) or weight-adjusted dalteparin for 48 hours.

If tenecteplase is not available the alternatives are:
- Streptokinase 1.5 mu/h (used in the elderly, less intracranial haemorrhage)
- Alteplase (rt-PA)
    - 15 mg i.v. bolus
    - Then 0.75 mg/kg (max 50 mg) infusion over 30 minutes
    - Then 0.5 mg/kg (max 35 mg) over the next hour (used in thromboembolic disease)
- Reteplase 10 mu i.v. bolus repeated at 30 minutes
    - Give 5000 units of heparin.

The contraindications to thrombolysis are given in **Table 13**.

Table 13. Contraindications to thrombolysis

- Aortic dissection (it is rare for a dissection to present as an anterior myocardial infarction)
- Previous cerebral haemorrhage
- Cerebral aneurysm, AV malformation, intracranial neoplasm
- Stroke (thromboembolic) within 6 months
- Internal bleeding (not menstruation)

Relative contraindications

- Blood pressure > 180/110 mmHg
  (give i.v. nitrates or a beta blocker)
- > 10 minutes of cardiopulmonary resuscitation or trauma in the last 4 weeks
- Surgery, biopsy or vessel puncture in last 3 weeks
- Pregnancy
- Active peptic ulcer disease

Pitfalls of thrombolysis

Remember:
- Very late thrombolysis offers only minimal benefit; this should be balanced against the risks
- Not every acute myocardial infarction should be thrombolysed. The clinical trials often excluded the elderly and other complex patient groups. It is not wrong to manage conservatively an uncomplicated inferior myocardial infarction in a 90-year-old patient with other co-morbid factors that put them at haemorrhagic risk.

Failed thrombolysis

Remember:
- Thrombolysis results in epicardial vessel patency in about 60–75% of patients, but normal capillary perfusion in 40–50% of patients
- Most clinicians use the ECG as a guide, with higher than 50% resolution in ST segment elevation at 90 minutes post-thrombolysis being considered successful therapy
- Reperfusion arrhythmias are also a good indication
- Failure of thrombolysis at 2 hours is associated with a 30-day mortality of 15%.

The options are:
- Rescue PCI
- Repeat thrombolysis
- Medical treatment.

Rescue angioplasty

You should discuss rescue angioplasty with a consultant, especially for large, anterior myocardial infarction or if there is haemodynamic compromise. Rescue angioplasty is less likely to achieve target vessel patency than is primary angioplasty. It should be performed within 8–12 hours to have a significant benefit, and ideally as soon as possible.

Repeat thrombolysis

With repeat thrombolysis there is:
- No mortality benefit
- Some improvement in left ventricular function
- Double the risk of intracerebral haemorrhage.

You should therefore consider it only if rescue angioplasty is not available and a substantial amount of myocardium is at risk.

SECONDARY TREATMENT ON THE CORONARY CARE UNIT
Beta blockers

Use:
- Atenolol 50 mg for men
- Atenolol 25 mg for small women.

Take care in patients with:
- Asthma
- AV block
- Left ventricular failure.

If any doubt exists use metoprolol 12.5 tds titrated up accordingly. If this is well tolerated, switch to atenolol because compliance is better with once-daily treatment.

Statins

The principle of statin treatment is to start high and reassess. Statins are indicated for all patients with ACS, even those with a normal baseline cholesterol. Our protocol is as follows:
- Give 40 mg of simvastatin or equivalent
- Reassess cholesterol at 3 months
- Aim for a total cholesterol of < 4.5 mmol/l and a low-density lipoprotein cholesterol of < 2.5 mmol/l
- Reduce the dose of simvastatin (20 mg) if the patient is also on warfarin or amiodarone (see Chapter 14).

Eplerenone

This selective aldosterone receptor antagonist has recently been licensed for patients post myocardial infarction with heart failure, and can be given 3–14 days post myocardial infarction. The European Society of Cardiology has recently included it in its guidelines. Ideally, suitable patients would already be on an ACE inhibitor and beta blocker. Initially give 25 mg once daily and titrate to 50 mg once daily within 1 month.

ACE inhibitors

ACE inhibitors are now standard treatment and should be given to all patients with acute myocardial infarction, even if they are normotensive. They are thought to reduce readmissions for heart failure, reinfarction and the need for revascularisation.

Dosages are as follows:
- Perindopril 2 mg, 4 mg, 8 mg
- Ramipril 1.25 mg, 2.5 mg, 5 mg, 10 mg.

Insulin

For patients with new or established diabetes or with a glucose level > 11.0 mmol/l on admission we prescribe:
- 50 units of Actrapid in 50 ml of 0.9% NaCl adjusted to a sliding scale
- 5% dextrose 30 ml/h.

Aim for a target blood glucose of 5.0–10.0 mmol/l.

Dosages of insulin are given in **Table 14**. Patients who need a continuous insulin infusion to maintain their blood sugar level should go home with subcutaneous insulin. The diabetic nurses should be fully involved in this process, but a good starting point is:
- Mixtard 30/70 0.5 units/kg in two divided doses (2/3 given in the morning, 1/3 given with the evening meal).

Table 14. Administering intravenous insulin

Blood glucose (mmol/l)	Insulin (ml/h)
> 20.0	4.0
15.1–20.0	3.0
10.1–15.0	2.0
5.0–10.0	1.0
< 5.0	0.5
< 3.0	Stop temporarily

Anti-anginal agents

These have no real role in the management of acute myocardial infarction. If there is evidence of ongoing cardiac chest pain then revascularisation is indicated. They may be used for interim stabilisation or for patients not suitable for revascularisation. They have been discussed in Chapter 1.

chapter 5

Heart failure

Nick Fisher
Janet Lock
Hayley Pryse-Hawkins

MANAGING ACUTE PULMONARY OEDEMA

The steps to take when managing patients with acute pulmonary oedema are as follows.

First things first

- Sit the patient up
- Give maximum oxygen (ball hitting the top) via a Venturi mask
- Give furosemide 80 mg stat i.v.
- Give diamorphine 2.5 mg (with metoclopramide 10 mg)
- Do a chest X-ray (to make sure the patient really has pulmonary oedema).

Find out why it has happened

- History: get the patient's previous notes and check for known heart failure; did they receive 6 l of fluid? Are they anuric? etc
- ECG: look for ischaemia and arrhythmia
- Echocardiograph: look for aortic stenosis, aortic regurgitation, mitral regurgitation and, of course, left ventricular function
- Bloods: order a full blood count (FBC), urea and electrolytes (U&Es), troponin level.

Find out how bad it is

- Measure arterial blood gas
- Catheterise the patient for urine output.

If you are still having trouble

- Give another 40 mg furosemide i.v.
- If the patient's blood pressure is > 100 mmHg start GTN infusion 2–10 mg/h i.v.
- Start continuous positive airways pressure.

Things to consider

- Dopamine is a good diuretic, but it is not necessarily better than furosemide. It is given at 2.5–5.0 µg/kg/min
- Ischaemic patients will benefit from a balloon pump if they are not responding quickly, and especially if they are hypotensive
- Patients with poor urine output (often with known renal insufficiency) can be offloaded with haemofiltration
- Ventilation is the last, but effective, resort
- Two minds are better than one. Ask for help.

MANAGING CHRONIC HEART FAILURE

Remember that heart failure is not a benign condition. Some 50% of patients with heart failure die within 4 years, and within 1 year if the condition is severe. You should therefore consider these patients for palliative care.

Determine the symptoms and signs

When assessing the patient's signs and symptoms, remember to use the New York Heart Association (NYHA) classification of heart failure (**Table 15**).

Investigations

Obtain the following tests.

- ECG: note Q waves, left bundle branch block, left ventricular hypertrophy, atrial fibrillation, PR interval (if normal, chronic heart failure is less likely)
- Chest X-ray: don't forget cardiothoracic ratio > 50%
- Bloods: FBC, liver function tests, U&Es, C-reactive protein, thyroid function tests, glucose, cardiac enzymes (if acute) and brain natriuretic peptide (if available)

Table 15. New York Heart Association classification of heart failure

Classification	Description	Notes
Class I	No limitation	Ordinary physical activity does not cause undue fatigue, dyspnoea or palpitations
Class II	Slight limitation of physical activity	Such patients are comfortable at rest. Ordinary physical activity results in fatigue, palpitations, dyspnoea or angina
Class III	Marked limitation of physical activity	Although patients are comfortable at rest, less than ordinary activity will lead to symptoms. Patients cannot climb a flight of stairs
Class IV	Inability to carry on any physical activity without discomfort	Symptoms of congestive failure are present even at rest. Patients experience increased discomfort with any physical activity

- Echocardiogram: record the ejection fraction (normal $\geq 55\%$), chamber dimensions, wall motion defects, valvular function, pulmonary artery pressure from tricuspid regurgitation.

Determine the aetiology and precipitating exacerbating features

Most cases of chronic heart failure will be due to ischaemic heart disease, but you should also consider:

- Arrhythmias
- Valve dysfunction
- Cardiomyopathy
- Anaemia
- Pericardial disease
- Pulmonary embolism
- Infection
- Thyroid disease
- Drugs.

If you have not accurately determined the extent of ischaemic heart disease, you need to do so. If the patient is symptomatic and an exercise tolerance test is likely to yield little information (especially if there is a starting abnormal ECG), then get a nuclear perfusion scan. If this shows significant reversible ischaemia, the next step is angiography with a view to revascularisation.

Cardiac MRI
This is worth considering if offered by your hospital. It will give you the following information:
- Chamber size, function and volume
- Cardiac mass
- Valvular function.

Using gadolinium (offered in some centres) it is possible to determine myocardial perfusion, and late opacification indicates fibrosis or infarction.

Myocardial oxygen consumption (MVO_2)
This test is used to stratify patients with severe heart failure for transplantation or left ventricular assist devices.

Advising the patient
Weight
Patients should weigh themselves daily. Sudden weight gain can be the first warning of problems. Patients should report an increase of more than 4 lb (2.4 kg) in one week, paroxysmal nocturnal dyspnoea or increased oedema.

Overweight patients (due to fat) need to lose weight. However, nutrition is important in patients with severe chronic heart failure; about half of patients with heart failure will become malnourished (cardiac cachexia).

Exercise
You should encourage patients to exercise, or to attend a specific training programme.

Diet

This should be balanced and healthy. Patients should assess and minimise their salt intake and avoid drinking more than 4 pints of fluid per day.

Stop smoking

You should encourage patients to stop smoking. Other risk factors are given in **Table 16**.

Table 16. Chronic heart failure: other risk factors

Advise patients to avoid:
• High altitudes
• Long-haul flights
• Drugs
   ◦ Non-steroidal anti-inflammatory drugs
   ◦ Effervescent preparations (e.g. soluble paracetamol) because they often contain high levels of sodium
   ◦ Calcium antagonists
   ◦ Tricyclic antidepressants
   ◦ Steroids
   ◦ Lithium

Drug treatment

Before you reach for the prescription pad, check whether you have tackled ischaemia, alcohol, drugs, thyroid disease and lifestyle.

Titrating drugs is essential for optimum management, and it is important that you ensure this happens. If you see a patient a year later and they are still receiving 2.5 mg of lisinopril, 3.125 mg of carvedilol and 10 mg of simvastatin, and they have a cholesterol level of 8.0 mmol/l, you have failed to treat them properly.

Add the following drugs in this order:
• ACE inhibitor (titrated to optimum dose)
• If symptomatic, add a diuretic

- Once symptoms are under control add a beta blocker (titrated to optimum dose)
- If symptoms persist, add spironolactone (class III–IV).

ACE inhibitors

Doses are as follows:
- Lisinopril: 2.5 mg titrated to 20 mg (in 2.5 mg stages)
- Ramipril: 2.5 mg titrated to 10 mg od
- Perindopril: 2 mg titrated to 4 mg.

The advantage of lisinopril and ramipril is that they allow slow titration when heart failure is severe or when there are complicating factors, such as renal dysfunction. The advantage of perindopril is that in mild heart failure it can be given in an outpatient clinic as a single 2 mg starting dose and then a 4 mg maintenance dose, if well tolerated. In a two-step process the patient will be on the target dose in 48 hours.

Start an ACE inhibitor only if:
- Serum creatinine is < 250 μmol/l (< 200 μmol/l if in outpatients)
- Potassium is < 5.5 mmol/l **AND**
- Systolic blood pressure is < 90 mmHg (> 100 mmHg and asymptomatic in outpatients).

Otherwise, investigate and manage with an aim to introduce an ACE inhibitor. Other points to remember are given in **Table 17**.

Diuretics

Doses are as follows:
- Furosemide: 20–40 mg initially (250–500 mg in divided doses in severe cases)
- Bumetanide: 0.5–1.0 mg initially (5–10 mg in divided doses in severe cases).

Patients on a diuretic should also be given an ACE inhibitor. If there is an insufficient response:

- First increase the dose
- Then add a thiazide
- Then switch to twice daily
- Then consider metolazone.

Thiazide diuretics are less effective if the glomerular filtration rate falls below 30 ml/min, which is not uncommon in elderly patients with heart failure. In severe heart failure thiazides have a synergistic effect with loop diuretics, so adding a thiazide is preferable to simply increasing the dose of a single loop diuretic.

Remember that the bowel will also be affected by oedema. This will lead to decreased oral absorption in severe heart failure (NYHA class IV).

Bumetanide
Remember:
- This is better absorbed from the oedematous gut
- Beware of possible glucose intolerance
- 1 mg is roughly equivalent to 40 mg of furosemide.

Amiloride

The only place for this drug is in the setting of severe heart failure and hypokalaemia despite an ACE inhibitor, loop diuretic and low-dose spironolactone (potassium supplements are less effective in these settings). The dose is 2.5 mg od.

Metolazone

You should add metolazone to a loop diuretic in patients with resistant oedema. The dose is 2.5–5 mg od. It can cause extensive diuresis so should be used with caution. Therefore, monitor sodium and potassium carefully. Some patients are able to take metolazone on a prn basis and are very good at self-controlling their heart failure.

Note that patients taking diuretics should ideally be monitoring their weight daily or at least three times a week. You should advise them to report any decrease or increase in weight. They should have blood checks for U&Es every 6 months, and more frequently if their doses need to be altered frequently.

When starting metolazone and spironolactone, check urea and electrolytes within 4–10 days.

Beta blockers

Doses are as follows:
- Bisoprolol: start with 1.25 mg daily, then add 1.25 mg every 2 weeks until 5 mg, then 2.5 mg monthly until 10 mg
- Carvedilol: start with 3.125 mg bd, then double the dose every 2–4 weeks until 25 mg bd or 50 mg bd if > 85 kg.

Bisoprolol and carvedilol have been shown to be beneficial in heart failure. On a practical level, carvedilol has a gentle titration curve, which helps with compliance.

Remember the importance of titration. Other points to consider are as follows:
- Before you start make sure the patient is on an ACE inhibitor and has no significant fluid retention

- The patient should be stable, with no acute exacerbation in the past month
- The patient should be compliant; confusion leads to impaired tolerance and reduces success
- Don't forget to ask about asthma
- Be very cautious if the blood pressure is < 100 mmHg systolic or if the pulse rate is < 50 bpm. If in doubt, admit the patient to start treatment
- Advise patients that they are likely to feel worse before they feel better, so they should try to stick with their treatment
- Diabetes can impair the stability of blood sugar control, and may impair awareness of altering blood sugar levels.

Spironolactone

Points to remember when prescribing spironolactone are as follows:
- Give 25 mg od, and if tolerated increase to 50 mg od
- Add spironolactone if the patient has severe failure (NYHA class III or IV)
- DO NOT give if potassium is > 5 mmol/l OR if creatinine is > 250 µmol/l
- Check potassium after 1 week
  - If it goes over 5 mmol/l, reduce the dose by half
  - If it goes over 5.5 mmol/l, STOP spironolactone
- If the patient's U&Es are stable after 1 month, increase to 50 mg od if the patient has not improved
- Painful gynaecomastia can occur in up to 10% of patients; you may need to stop the spironolactone or switch to eplerenone 25 mg od.

Eplerenone

This selective aldosterone receptor antagonist has recently been licensed for patients post myocardial infarction with heart failure, and can be given 3–14 days post myocardial infarction. The European Society of Cardiology has recently included it in its guidelines. Ideally, suitable patients would already be on an ACE inhibitor and beta blocker. Initially give 25 mg once daily and titrate to 50 mg once daily within 1 month. Remember, this drug does not have the side effects of gynaecomastia and breast pain.

Other treatments
Digoxin
Digoxin is used more frequently in the US than in the UK and has not been shown to reduce mortality, but it does seem to reduce symptoms. We don't routinely use it. It can reduce hospital admissions in severe, unstable patients.

Dopamine
Dopamine is given intravenously via a central line (2.5–5.0 µg/kg/min). It produces a good diuresis and can be used in severe heart failure to bail you out when furosemide does not seem to be working. Remember, just because you have created an increase in diuresis you have not improved renal function. You should therefore use dopamine only for the short-term management of haemodynamic disturbances.

Pacemakers
Pacemakers should be used for appropriate bradycardia or heart block as with any other condition. Biventricular pacing is coming into vogue, but your department may not offer this. It currently appears to benefit people with NYHA class III or IV heart failure that is refractory to normal medical treatment, left bundle branch block and a QRS complex > 120 ms.

Correcting anaemia
Patients with a haemoglobin level of < 11 g/dl should be considered for further investigation and treatment (iron and erythropoietin). Implantable cardioverter defibrillators are discussed in Chapter 11 and heart transplantation is discussed in Chapter 12.

THE HEART FAILURE NURSE

Consider referring all patients with objective evidence of heart failure to the heart failure nurse. Many hospitals also hold a heart failure support group each month for patients and relatives. Ask the clinic nurses for details.

Patients that you should definitely refer are given in **Table 18**. Try, whenever possible, to integrate patients into the community or primary care for follow-up. All patients with heart failure should be reviewed six monthly. This does not need to be done by a doctor or in a hospital setting, but patients should be aware of this.

Table 18. The heart failure nurse: who to refer

- New diagnosis of heart failure
- Patients who have been admitted to hospital more than twice for decompensated heart failure in the past 12 months
- Patients requiring initiation and titration of beta blockers. If they are started on a beta blocker in the clinic you should give them contact details for the heart failure nurse (don't forget to send them a copy of the clinic letter; ask the secretary to email the letter so they get it quickly)
- Unstable patients in the community needing frequent diuretic adjustments
- Patients needing cardiac rehabilitation or exercise training
- Patients needing in-depth lifestyle advice and modification
- Patients needing an assessment for left ventricular assist devices and/or transplantation (don't forget the transplant sister)
- Patients needing palliative or end-stage care

The contact details for my heart failure nurse are:

Tel: _____

Fax: _____

Email: _____

chapter 6

Hypertension

Nick Fisher
Janet Lock

INTRODUCTION

If you don't think blood pressure is important or if you think it's a bit below you as a cardiologist, ask yourself how much atheroma you have ever seen in a pulmonary artery. If you have moderate hypertension you have a higher chance of dying from a myocardial infarction than of dying from a stroke. In addition, hypertension is now second only to ischaemic heart disease as a cause of heart failure.

Interested now? Remember that systolic blood pressure rises throughout life, but diastolic hypertension is maximal by age 50–59 years. Isolated systolic hypertension is the biggest killer.

Guidelines

In June 2003, the European Society of Cardiology released new guidelines that unusually differed from US guidelines released earlier in the year (Seventh Report of the Joint National Committee on Prevention Detection, Evaluation and Treatment of High Blood Pressure).[2, 3] In 2004, new guidelines from the British Hypertension Society mirrored the European Society of Cardiology guidelines.[4]

There are two main differences between the European and US guidelines:

- Definition of hypertension – the US guidelines classify a systolic blood pressure of 120–139 mmHg and a diastolic blood pressure of 80–89 mmHg as 'pre hypertension'. The Europeans classify these levels as 'high normal'

- Treatment – the ALLHAT study[5] indicated that diuretics either alone or in combination with other agents should be first-line drugs of choice. The Europeans take the line that all antihypertensive agents can be considered as first-line therapy. This seems to make more sense. It appears that the main way that antihypertensive agents produce a benefit is by reducing blood pressure. It seems sensible, therefore, to achieve this objective and then consider whether there are any additional advantages to be used from your choice of agent. For example, if I had diabetes I would prefer an ACE inhibitor or angiotensin II receptor blocker for my hypertension.

IS IT HYPERTENSION?

First, you should establish whether your patient is hypertensive. Remember that labelling a patient as 'hypertensive' may have a significant psychological and socioeconomic effect.

Always have a well-documented series of measurements taken at different times of the day over 2–3 months with the correct sized cuff. *Always* measure blood pressure in both arms and make sure there is no radio-femoral delay (coarctation of the aorta).

24-hour ambulatory blood-pressure monitoring

If you are suspicious that the patient has significant white-coat hypertension or if the figures don't quite fit the patient (especially in the young), arrange a 24-hour ambulatory blood-pressure test. Don't just look at the 24-hour average of the results. Most blood pressure guidelines are based on daytime readings (rather than their average), which tend to be more representative.

Look for:
- Early morning peaks (when most myocardial infarctions occur)
- Absence of the normal night-time low.

Although a daytime average may be normal, a significant number of very high (> 160/100 mmHg) readings without a good reason (such as running for a bus) should not pass you unnoticed. Equally, a wide pulse pressure is a potent indicator of cardiovascular risk, i.e. a blood pressure of 150/85 mmHg is more significant than one of 150/95 mmHg.

Symptoms

Despite patients' convictions that they are aware of when their blood pressure is raised, there is little real association between symptoms and blood pressure. One exception is an early morning occipital headache radiating to the front that eases off during the day. Also, remember that a phaeochromocytoma can cause headache, sweating and palpitations (sometimes with pallor or feelings of impending doom).

Ask about:
- Family history
- Alcohol intake (don't take 'sociably' as an answer – nail the patient down to an amount and work out the exact units; ask about binge drinking)
- Drugs – cocaine, steroids (especially in body builders), non-steroidal anti-inflammatory drugs (NSAIDs), oral contraceptives and venlafaxine
- Salt intake
- Smoking
- Symptoms of pulmonary oedema (be aware of recurrent flash pulmonary oedema of renal artery stenosis)
- Ischaemic heart disease
- Diabetes
- Connective tissue disease.

Points not to miss are given in **Table 19**.

Table 19. Diagnosing hypertension: what not to miss	
Feature	**Notes**
Coarctation	R/R R/F delay. Large, well-built torso with matchstick legs
Bruit of renal artery stenosis	
Retinal disease	Don't blag it. If you have 4-year-old batteries in your ophthalmoscope and a sunny room with no curtains, find better equipment and move to another room or refer to the ophthalmologist for a proper look through a dilated pupil. **Don't miss retinal disease secondary to hypertension**
Urine dipstick results	If blood and protein are present send samples for microscopy, culture and sensitivity, asking the lab to look out especially for granular or cellular casts indicative of underlying renal disease

Investigations

FBC, U&Es

Remember to look for renal failure, anaemia, polycythaemia and low potassium (occurs with Conn's). If connective tissue disease or renal pathology is on your mind then check erythrocyte sedimentation rate, C-reactive protein and autoantibodies.

ECG

Check for:

- R wave in V5/6
- S wave in V1/2 > 25 mm
- A combination of the R/S > 35 mm.

Young, thin and athletic people have higher voltages, while obese people have lower ones. Voltages in non-white patients are also less specific.

As you have probably guessed, diagnosing left ventricular hypertrophy by voltage is pretty unreliable. However, left ventricular hypertrophy diagnosed by voltage *and* repolarisation changes (often called strain) has as poor a prognosis as a previous myocardial infarction. If repolarisation changes are present, look at the echocardiogram to make sure it's not due to hypertrophic cardiomyopathy.

Chest X-ray
Note any rib notching (coarctation).

Renal ultrasound/MRI
This will pick up:
- Polycystic kidneys
- Obstructive uropathy
- Reduction in kidney size or inequality of more than 1.5 cm
- Parenchymal thinning suggestive of chronic renal disease.

A significant inequality in size should alert you to renal artery stenosis, and you should book an MR angiogram.

24-hour urine
This is to detect vanillylmandelic acid. Results twice that of normal are often diagnostic for phaeochromocytoma. One collection should be enough. Patients with an elevated level should be referred to an endocrinologist who will probably organise plasma noradrenaline.

Echocardiogram
Note left ventricle dimensions, which are normally measured in the parasternal long axis in end diastole. Measurements are taken from leading edge to leading edge beyond the tips of the mitral valve. They are rather subjective and operator dependent. Check for regional hypertrophy outside the measured area. In short, don't hang your hat on measurements; if in doubt, get the tape out and have a look.

Table 20. Normal left ventricle dimensions	
Septum:	< 13 mm in men < 12 mm in women
Posterior wall:	< 12 mm in men < 11 mm in women

Normal values are shown in **Table 20**.

Cardiac MRI

The images obtained with cardiac MRI allow a more accurate assessment of left ventricle morphology, function and mass. To date there are no significant studies linking MRI data to outcome, but it is likely to be only a matter of time.

WHO TO TREAT

Note that the information in this section is not relevant for pregnant women.

You should treat:
- Anyone with a blood pressure > 160/100 mmHg
- Anyone with a blood pressure > 140/90 mmHg with:
  - Ischaemic heart disease
  - Diabetes
  - Any indication of end-organ damage or
  - Coronary heart disease (CHD) risk ≥ 20% over 10 years.

You should not treat anyone with a blood pressure < 135/85 mmHg.

Values between 140/90 mmHg and 160/100 mmHg are not so black and white, and depend on other risk factors. If the patient's blood pressure is > 140/90 mmHg and the patient has risk factors then you should treat them. Remember, you don't have to rush straight into pharmacological treatment, especially if there are no risk factors. Try giving weight loss, alcohol reduction and dietary changes a go first.

TREATMENT TARGETS

You should reduce the blood pressure to at least 150/90 mmHg, aiming for a target of 140/85 mmHg. If the patient has diabetes, an ideal level would be 140/80 mmHg.

Less than 10% of surveys show that patients have reached the target; don't let your management contribute to this statistic.

PATIENT ADVICE

Advise patients to:

- Lose weight – a 1 kg increase in weight is associated with a 1 mmHg increase in systolic blood pressure
- Exercise – 30 minutes a day of aerobic exercise can reduce blood pressure by 4–9 mmHg
- Reduce or avoid alcohol – this is the most common treatable cause of resistant hypertension (limit to 21 units for men, 14 units for women)
- Reduce salt intake
- Become a vegetarian – if a patient is adamant that they don't want to take drugs then they could try being a vegetarian; vegetarians have lower blood pressures at all ages than omnivores
- Stop smoking.

DRUG TREATMENT

Unless the patient's blood pressure is > 160/110 mmHg, make sure you have eliminated all treatable causes (i.e. diagnosed essential hypertension) and offer them a chance to lose weight and change their lifestyle before you commit them lifelong to drugs. Set an agreed timeframe, for example 3 months to try these measures. If they haven't made any significant difference in this time bite the bullet and start drug treatment.

Before you agonise over which is the best drug, remember that getting the blood pressure down is more important than the choice of drug. Traditionally, people have used the AB/CD rule.

- White patients younger than 55 years tend to have a high renin vasoconstrictor condition, which is better suited to ACE inhibitors and beta blockers (AB)

- African Caribbean and white patients older than 55 years tend to have low renin volume-dependent hypertension, which is more suited to calcium antagonists and diuretics (CD).

This has been questioned by the recent ASCOT study,[6] which clearly indicated that amlodipine and perindopril were superior to atenolol and a diuretic. It would therefore seem wise to steer away from atenolol unless there are other indications, such as arrhythmias or ischaemic heart disease.

In summary, drug options are:
- ACE inhibitors or angiotensin II receptor blockers
- Beta blockers
- Calcium antagonists
- Diuretics.

If you are still having trouble

If treatment is not working:
- Make sure the patient really has reduced their alcohol intake
- Check again that renal artery stenosis was eliminated
- Consider Conn's syndrome because many patients have a normal serum potassium despite having raised aldosterone to renin ratios. Very few will actually have an adenoma. If you can't get aldosterone to renin ratios, then give a trial with spironolactone (1 mg/kg to the nearest 25 mg).

Then add:
- A beta blocker
- A centrally acting antihypertensive.

Remember that managing hypertension is just part of the secondary prevention of CHD. Patients should therefore receive statins if indicated by the CHD risk tables (found at the back of the *British National Formulary*). They should also receive aspirin if their blood pressure is controlled, they are age 50 years or older or have evidence of end-organ damage.

Hyperlipidaemia

Nick Fisher
Janet Lock

PRIMARY PREVENTION

Remember:

- Because cholesterol levels can vary slightly it is worth repeating borderline cases about 1 month apart
- Total cholesterol and high-density lipoprotein (HDL) can be determined from a non-fasting blood sample
- Low-density lipoprotein (LDL) and triglycerides require a fasting blood sample
- Before committing someone to lifelong statin therapy, check the baseline fasting lipid profile, creatinine kinase and liver enzymes
- Use the guidelines set out in the government's national service framework for CHD.[7]

HDL, LDL and the ratios

The use and relevance of cholesterol subdivisions and ratios can be confusing. An acceptable approach is to:

- Check total cholesterol is < 4.0 mmol/l (and if you stop here you will be doing well!)
- If a full screen is available, then
  - Total cholesterol:HDL ratio should be < 4.0 mmol/l
  - LDL should be < 2.5 mmol/l.

There really are no guidelines for HDL and triglycerides, but there is an added risk of CHD if:

- Fasting triglycerides are > 1.7 mmol/l (especially in people with diabetes)
- HDL is < 1 mmol/l.

Treatment

Give a statin to:
- Patients with a CHD risk of $\geq$ 30% over 10 years
- Anyone with a cholesterol of > 7.5 mmol/l (also screen for familial hyperlipidaemia)
- Anyone with diabetes.

Have a low threshold with Asian people and patients with a CHD score $\geq$ 15% over 10 years.

One treatment approach is as follows:
- Start patients on 20 mg of simvastatin and increase to 40 mg if repeat cholesterols are not < 5 mmol/l
- If 40 mg of simvastatin is not effective switch to atorvastatin 20 mg *or* add ezetimibe
- If 40 mg atorvastatin (plus ezetimibe if not effective) titrate up to 80 mg or, if the patient is not Asian/Oriental, switch to rosuvastatin, remembering to start at 10 mg and wait a month before increasing to 20 mg.

Treatment target

Reduce cholesterol below 5 mmol/l. (A 25% reduction is also considered to be satisfactory, but we would aim for < 5 mmol/l.)

Next steps

Within 3 months check:
- Cholesterol
- Creatinine kinase
- Liver enzymes.

Repeat these at 6 months and at 1 year. From then on repeat annually.

SECONDARY PREVENTION

All patients who have had a myocardial infarction should receive a statin. Aim for a total cholesterol of ≤ 4 mmol/l. The treatment approach for primary prevention is also appropriate here.

Remember:

- Serum transaminase concentrations can transiently rise and statins should be stopped if they are persistently three times higher than reference values
- Myopathy is a rare but significant complication. Discontinue statins if creatinine kinase is five times higher than normal levels
- Simvastatin potentiates the effect of warfarin and often needs about a 30% decrease in the warfarin dose
- Avoid statins in pregnancy and when breast feeding
- Simvastatin (and to a lesser extent atorvastatin) is particularly sensitive to drug interactions (see Chapter 14). Substances that increase its levels are given in **Table 21**.

Table 21. Drug interactions with simvastatin and atorvastatin

Drug or substance	Recommendation
• Azole antifungals • Macrolides • HIV protease inhibitors	Avoid simvastatin; exercise caution with atorvastatin; stop statin during therapy and for two days after therapy
• Ciclosporin • Fibrates	Do not exceed simvastatin 10 mg; exercise caution with atorvastatin
• Verapamil • Amiodarone	Do not exceed simvastatin 20 mg; exercise caution with atorvastatin
• Diltiazem	Do not exceed simvastatin 40 mg
• Grapefruit juice	Avoid simvastatin; avoid > 200 ml with atorvastatin

Chronic valvular heart disease

Nick Fisher
Derek Gibson

INTRODUCTION

This chapter is based on the American Heart Association guide-lines.[8]

Echocardiograms

Would you refer yourself for a valve replacement without having seen your own echocardiogram? I guess not, so you shouldn't do so with your patients. Try not to make a decision based on a scan you haven't seen. Ask yourself:

- Were the views good?
- What was the ventricular function really like?
- Was the Doppler accurately aligned?
- Was anything missed?
- Who did the report?

One of the biggest crimes with echocardiography is to ignore what you see. Never see an echocardiogram that looks worse than the last and simply order another one in 6 months' time, in the hope that someone else will see the patient and make a decision (the doctor who ordered the last scan may have done that already).

Cardiothoracic surgeons

There is nothing worse than to 'sit on' a patient with steadily decreasing left ventricular function for fear of approaching a sur-geon. Any surgeon worth their salt won't mind discussing a patient with you, and this open dialogue is undoubtedly the best way to manage patients that may be candidates for valve repair or replacement. You will quickly learn what factors the surgeon places more importance on than you do. Patients rarely pigeon-hole themselves as nicely as we would wish, and a combined approach to their management is best.

AORTIC STENOSIS

If you come across a patient with aortic stenosis you need to make sure you know:

- How symptomatic they are
- What the echocardiogram shows
- When to consider surgery.

As always, you must remember antibiotic prophylaxis.

Signs and symptoms

Significant symptoms are:

- Angina
- Dyspnoea
- Syncope.

The development of these symptoms marks a critical point in the natural history of aortic stenosis. If you ignore them in a patient with significant disease, they could be dead within 3 years.

Document clearly the patient's current level of activity. They may still have no breathlessness because they have stopped trying to walk very far.

Echocardiogram

You need to look for:

- The peak gradient across the valve (moderate aortic stenosis > 50 mmHg; and severe aortic stenosis > 80 mmHg).
  Remember: peak gradient = 4 x (velocity^2). In general, if the

velocity is > 4 m/s (64 mmHg) then the patient has significant disease. Remember that aortic regurgitation will cause you to overestimate the gradient and mitral regurgitation to underestimate it. This is why you should also look at the valve area

- Ventricular function and ejection fraction
- Increasing left atrial pressure
- Evidence of pulmonary hypertension (if the ventricular function falls off so will the gradient, and the patient is getting worse rather than better)
- The valve area. Find out whether this is measured by planimetry or derived from the continuity equation. Planimetry (drawing around the hole) of a calcified aortic valve is not very accurate, so you should ignore this and try to look for an area obtained by the continuity equation.

Remember:
- Normal aortic valve = 3–4 cm^2
- Moderate aortic stenosis = 0.6–1.0 cm^2
- Severe aortic stenosis = < 0.6 cm^2.

Follow-up

Follow up patients (with an echocardiogram) as follows:
- Asymptomatic patients with mild-to-moderate disease at 2 years
- Asymptomatic patients with severe disease at 1 year.

Review patients who experience a change in symptom severity or values every 6 months *and* give them open access if their symptoms deteriorate.

Follow-up should also include an annual ECG and chest X-ray:
- ECG – look for QRS elongation and T-wave inversion, which is a good sign of left ventricle disease
- Chest X-ray – look for signs of pulmonary congestion and increasing cardiothoracic ratio.

Aortic valve replacement

Consider aortic valve replacement in:

- Symptomatic patients with severe aortic stenosis
- Patients with severe or moderate aortic stenosis who need a coronary artery bypass graft (CABG) or aortic surgery
- Asymptomatic patients with severe aortic stenosis *and*
  - Left ventricular systolic dysfunction (only need a gradient of > 40 mmHg)
  - An abnormal response to exercise (e.g. hypotension)
  - Ventricular tachycardia
- Patients whose valve area is < 0.6 cm²
- Patients with marked or excessive left ventricular hypertrophy (> 15 mm).

Cardiac catheterisation

No patient or surgeon will thank you if you decide that a CABG is needed a year after an aortic valve replacement. Unless you have a young patient with absolutely no risk of ischaemic heart disease you should determine the state of the coronary arteries before the valve replacement. If the need for valve replacement is unequivocal there is no need to cross the valve.

In some cases, if the diagnosis is in doubt a surgeon may ask for a withdrawal gradient. Remember that the peak echocardiogram gradient corresponds to the maximum instantaneous gradient, not the peak to peak gradient measured during a catheterisation, which will be lower (**Figure 2**).

It is not 'cool' to spend 40 minutes worth of radiation crossing a very tight aortic valve, throwing off a few emboli while you're at it.

Medical treatment of inoperable cases

Take care not to reduce the preload excessively because this will reduce cardiac output and, therefore, systemic arterial pressure. However, if the patient is in failure you have no choice, so use diuretics and ACE inhibitors cautiously. Despite opinion to the contrary, there is evidence that ACE inhibitors are beneficial, and

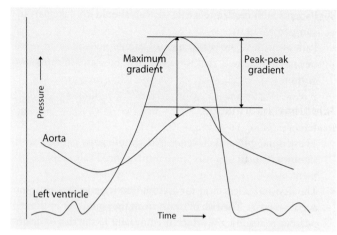

Figure 2. Example of left ventricular and aortic pressures measured with fluid-filled catheters in a patient with severe aortic stenosis. The maximum instantaneous gradient is greater than the peak to peak gradient, which is why catheter and echo values are not identical (because they are measuring different things).

no studies say that they are harmful. Use beta blockers with care (i.e. start with a low dose of metoprolol tds) for angina if nitrates are not working.

Remember that you should treat this condition medically only if the patient cannot have surgery. No patient is too ill for surgery if the illness is due to the stenosis. Correct this and you will remove the illness.

Patient advice

Patients should receive antibiotic prophylaxis for dental work or 'dirty procedures'. Advice about physical activity should be as follows:

- Asymptomatic patients and those with mild aortic stenosis can do whatever activities they like

- Patients with moderate aortic stenosis should not take part in competitive sport
- Patients with severe aortic stenosis should not engage in vigorous physical activity that will need large increases in cardiac output.

Additional information

Remember:

- There is unequivocal evidence that symptomatic patients with significant aortic stenosis (> 50 mmHg) need valve replacement
- The decision is less clear for asymptomatic patients with severe aortic stenosis. The risk of death from the condition in these patients is around 2%, which is equivalent to the risk of death from aortic valve replacement and the postoperative complications. If the valve is left too long, myocardial fibrosis and severe hypertrophy may be irreversible. Close (open access) monitoring is therefore needed to catch any deterioration in these patients. High-risk patients are rarely asymptomatic, but you need to be looking for it
- Never perform an exercise test on a patient with symptomatic or severe aortic stenosis. As an exception, some asymptomatic patients may undergo a test if symptoms or disease severity is in doubt, but you must be present during the test with one eye on the patient's blood pressure and pulse
- Patients with significant left ventricular dysfunction and a gradient < 30 mmHg don't do well with surgery
- Patients with asymptomatic aortic stenosis may undergo non-cardiac operations, but operative haemodynamics should be closely monitored
- QRS elongation is good evidence for left ventricular disease, as is T-wave inversion (therefore avoid digoxin if you can)
- Stentless valves are preferable, particularly if the pre-operative left ventricular disease is significant, because the stents themselves produce a degree of stenosis.

CHRONIC AORTIC REGURGITATION

It is important to emphasise that we are talking about regurgitation due to valvular pathology (e.g. bicuspid aortic valve) rather than pathology of the aortic root (e.g. Marfan's syndrome). In the latter case it may be the extent and rate of root dilatation that determine surgery.

Signs and symptoms

The most common symptoms are dyspnoea on exertion and decreased exercise tolerance. Symptoms are due to left ventricular dysfunction, not aortic valve disease. Other points to note are:

- If pulse pressure is > 50% systolic or > 70% diastolic the condition is unlikely to be severe
- If you really can hear an Austin flint murmur (a mid and late diastolic apical rumble) or demonstrate Duroziez's sign (systolic murmur heard over the femoral artery when compressed proximally, and diastolic murmur when compressed distally), the condition is likely to be severe.

Echocardiogram

Remember:

- Check the aortic root dimensions
- Look at the colour flow. You can't give it a number for future comparison or use it to make a decision about aortic valve replacement, but it quickly tells you whether the condition is likely to be significant or trivial. If the width of the colour flow is more than 60% of the outflow tract, the condition is significant
- The most significant measurement is end-systolic and end-diastolic dimensions (end systolic < end diastolic)
- Doppler alone is not sufficient, but it is very helpful if the degree of ventricular dilatation is out of proportion to the severity of regurgitation (e.g. due to ischaemic cardiomyopathy). Severe aortic regurgitation causes a pressure half-time of < 300 ms. Note that this is really a measure of the extent to

which left ventricular end-diastolic pressure approaches aortic diastolic pressure, and therefore the extent to which coronary flow may be compromised.

Medical treatment
Remember:
- Patients benefit from afterload reduction
- Give an ACE inhibitor (e.g. perindopril 2 mg titrated to 4 mg if tolerated after 24 hours)
- Nifedipine has the most documented benefit in severe cases (choose any long-acting drug).

Follow-up
Follow up patients (with an echocardiogram) as follows:
- Asymptomatic patients with mild-to-moderate disease at 2 years
- Asymptomatic patients with severe disease at 1 year.

Review patients who experience a change in symptom severity or values, or if the end-diastolic dimension is > 60 mm, every 6 months *and* give them open access if their symptoms deteriorate.

Always obtain a chest X-ray for pulmonary oedema and heart size, and an ECG for QRS duration.

Cardiac catheterisation
As with aortic stenosis, unless you have a young patient with absolutely no risk of ischaemic heart disease you need to determine the state of the coronary arteries before the aortic valve replacement. If there is any doubt, cross the valve to get a good ventriculogram. Also, inject another bolus into the root.

Aortic valve replacement
Consider aortic valve replacement in:
- Symptomatic patients (NYHA class III or IV)
- Patients with an ejection fraction < 25% normal or < 50% original

- Patients with an end-diastolic dimension > 75 mm or end-systolic dimension > 55 mm (reduce slightly in small patients)
- Patients undergoing CABG or aortic surgery.

If you can demonstrate increasing heart size on the echocardiogram or chest X-ray you should at least involve the surgeons in the decision-making process.

Patient advice

As with aortic stenosis, patients should receive antibiotic prophylaxis for dental work or dirty procedures. Asymptomatic patients can participate in sport, but isometric exercises (e.g. weight training) should be avoided.

Additional information

Remember:
- After an aortic valve replacement, a good predictor of subsequent left ventricular systolic function is the end-diastolic dimension, which declines significantly within the first week or two after the operation. In fact, 80% of overall reduction will occur by 2 weeks
- Review patients at 6 and 12 months, and then annually
- Continue with an ACE inhibitor unless left ventricular volume is normal
- Don't underestimate the complexity of the combination of chronic aortic regurgitation and separate left ventricular disease.

MITRAL STENOSIS

Mitral stenosis is a continuing lifelong disease usually consisting of a slow, stable course in the early years followed by progressive acceleration in later life.

Signs and symptoms

Patients can go for decades without symptoms, but when they occur they tend to be dyspnoea or pulmonary oedema, or due to an embolic event.

Symptoms on exertion are unlikely until:
- Valve area is < 2.5 cm² (normal mitral valve area = 4.0–5.0 cm²)
- Pulmonary arterial hypertension occurs
- Atrial fibrillation occurs.

Echocardiogram

The success of any conservative procedure (i.e. valvotomy or valvu-loplasty rather than mitral valve replacement) depends on:
- Mitral valve morphology and movement
- Leaflet mobility
- Mitral valve thickness
- Mitral valve calcification
- Presence of subvalvular fusion.

The appearance of commissures is also important when consider-ing intervention.

Document:
- Chamber dimensions and function, especially left atrium and right ventricle
- Mean transmural gradient using continuous wave Doppler
- Valve area – this can be derived from the diastolic pressure half-time (T) method (A_{MV} = 220/T, where T is measured in milliseconds) or the continuity equation. (This won't be accu-rate if left atrial or left ventricular compliance is abnormal or if there is mitral or aortic regurgitation, or if there has been a previous valvotomy.) Valve area can also be determined from planimetry of a 2D short axis view (only worthwhile if the valve is not calcified)
- Pulmonary artery pressure – this should be determined from any tricuspid regurgitation
- Severity of mitral and aortic regurgitation
- Organic tricuspid valve disease.

In asymptomatic patients, no further evaluation is needed if the valve area is > 1.5 cm² and the gradient is < 5 mmHg.

Follow-up
Patients should be followed up as follows:
- ECG and chest X-ray (left atrial size and pulmonary congestion) annually
- Echocardiogram every 5 years or if the patient becomes symptomatic.

Review patients who experience a change in symptom severity or values every 6 months *and* give them open access if their symptoms deteriorate. Remember that symptoms are your best guide to the progress of this condition. People do not die suddenly from mitral stenosis.

Cardiac catheterisation
Unless you have a young patient with absolutely no risk of ischaemic heart disease you need to determine the state of the coronary arteries before a mitral valve replacement.

In cases where the echocardiogram data do not fit the patient, left and right heart catheterisation should be carried out. You can use the Gorlin equation to calculate the mitral valve area. You can calculate the transmitral gradient by using the pulmonary artery wedge pressure as a substitute for left atrial pressure. However, this is often an overestimation even after correcting for phase delay. In addition, pulmonary artery pressure and resistance can be calculated.

Medical treatment
The problem is one of obstruction and, if possible, this should be removed. Atrial fibrillation in the presence of mitral valve disease carries a particularly high embolic risk; patients identified as developing atrial fibrillation should receive immediate anticoagulation with heparin while starting warfarin therapy.

Patient advice
Patients should receive antibiotic prophylaxis for dental work or dirty procedures. Advice about physical activity should be as follows:

- Asymptomatic patients and those with mild mitral stenosis can do whatever activities they like
- Low-level cardiovascular exercise is fine, but repeated vigorous exercise should not be encouraged because of the associated repeated exercise-induced increases in pulmonary venous and arterial pressure.

Percutaneous balloon valvotomy

Valvotomy is best in patients with pliable, non-calcified valves with little or no sub-valvular fusion. There should not be any left atrial thrombus, moderate or severe mitral regurgitation, or aortic or tricuspid valve disease.

Patients should be considered for this procedure if they are:
- Symptomatic and the valve area is ≤ 1.5 cm^2 (gradient ≥ 5 mmHg)
- Asymptomatic and the valve area is ≤ 1.5 cm^2 in the presence of pulmonary hypertension (pulmonary artery pressure > 50 mmHg at rest) or new-onset atrial fibrillation
- Asymptomatic and considering pregnancy.

Mitral valve replacement

Mitral valve replacement (instead of repair) is indicated:
- When percutaneous valvotomy is unavailable
- For patients with non-pliable calcified valves who otherwise fit the criteria above.

Mitral valve prolapse

This needs a mention because it is the most common form of valvular heart disease, affecting up to 6% of the population.

Echocardiogram

Look for:
- M mode: ≥ 2 mm posterior displacement of a leaflet, and holosystolic posterior 'hammocking' > 3 mm

- Parasternal long axis 2D: systolic displacement of at least one mitral leaflet.

Otherwise, assess as for mitral regurgitation.

Additional information

Remember:

- If there is no click or murmur, there is no mitral valve prolapse and no need for an echocardiogram
- As a group, the incidence of endocarditis is low but it is a serious complication. If you are aware of mitral valve prolapse you should advise antibiotic prophylaxis
- Some patients report a syndrome of palpitations (often with normal 24-hour tapes), atypical chest pain, dyspnoea and fatigue with no objective evidence, and neuropsychiatric symptoms. Reassurance and occasionally beta blockers are all that is needed, but be aware that these patients have often adopted the illness role and will transfer their affections to where they are most appreciated
- Follow-up is determined by the severity of the mitral regurgitation
- There is no embolic risk if the patient is in sinus rhythm.

CHRONIC MITRAL REGURGITATION
Signs and symptoms

Patients can remain asymptomatic for many years. It is important to establish and document baseline exercise tolerance so you can gauge the subtle onset of decreasing exercise tolerance and dyspnoea.

Echocardiogram

There are several Doppler methods for quantifying the severity of regurgitation, but none has been shown to predict clinical outcome. Colour flow is best used to differentiate the condition into mild, moderate and severe disease.

You need to know:
- Description of colour flow
- Ventricular function, dimensions (end systolic and end diastolic) and ejection fraction
- Left atrium dimensions
- Pulmonary artery pressure by tricuspid regurgitation.

Severe mitral regurgitation often follows chordal or papillary rupture or prosthetic failure.

Transoesophageal echocardiography
If a patient is symptomatic or has severe mitral regurgitation, transoesophageal echocardiography may be performed because repair may be an option. Using this method the leaflets are more easily visualised and the mechanism of regurgitation more accurately determined.

Often the pulmonary veins are assessed looking for flow reversal, which indicates severe mitral regurgitation. In reality there is little more to be gained over a good-quality transthoracic echocardiogram.

Follow-up
Patients should be followed up as follows:
- Asymptomatic patients with mild-to-moderate mitral regurgitation at 1 year (echocardiogram if symptomatic or if it is 5 years since the last one)
- Asymptomatic patients with severe mitral regurgitation every 6 months, with an echocardiogram.

Review patients who experience a change in symptom severity or values every 6 months *and* give them open access if their symptoms deteriorate.

Medical treatment
Treatment is not necessary for asymptomatic patients, while patients with symptoms need surgery. Treat other conditions (e.g. atrial fibrillation) in the usual way.

Cardiac catheterisation

Unless you have a young patient with absolutely no risk of ischaemic heart disease you need to determine the state of the coronary arteries before a mitral valve replacement.

In uncertain cases, cardiac catheterisation may provide further assessment of ventricular size and function as well as visualisation of the mitral regurgitation. A right heart catheter will give you pulmonary artery pressure and wedge pressure (left atrial pressure). The overall severity of mitral valve disease (stenotic or regurgitant) can be assessed from the difference between mean left atrial pressure and left ventricular end-diastolic pressure. In addition, the presence or absence of a large V wave in the pulmonary artery wedge pressure adds little to the overall picture.

Mitral valve repair or replacement

Patients undergo repair or replacement (with or without preservation of the mitral apparatus). Because the mitral apparatus is an integral part of the left ventricle and is essential for its normal shape, volume and function, it is important to preserve it if possible.

Valve calcification, rheumatic involvement and anterior leaflet involvement make repair less likely to succeed, whereas repair in patients with uncalcified posterior leaflet disease is most successful. In fact, a heavily calcified mitral ring makes surgery very difficult.

Mitral valve replacement is considered necessary when:
- Patients are symptomatic (regardless of function or dimensions)
- The end-systolic dimension is > 45 mm
- Left ventricular ejection fraction is < 60%.

Surgery is not recommended for asymptomatic patients with normal left ventricular function, unless it appears to be new onset due to chordal rupture or recent-onset atrial fibrillation.

Patient advice

Patients should receive antibiotic prophylaxis for dental work or dirty procedures. Advice about physical activity should be as follows:

- Asymptomatic patients with mild disease can do whatever activities they like
- Other patients should limit exercise to activities with low-to-moderate static cardiovascular demands.

VALVE REPLACEMENT

Be aware that manufacturers publish data outlining normal pressure gradients across their valves, which depends on size as well as make.

Ball valves

Starr–Edwards

These are not generally inserted any more, but there are still plenty about. Ball valves need more intense anticoagulation (INR: 3.0–4.5) than other types. Remember that a ball thrashing about can cause significant haemolytic anaemia.

Disc valves

Bjork–Shiley

These were introduced in 1969 and used a single tilting disc. The design was modified in the 1980s and, as a result, the retaining strut of some models was prone to fracture with terminal results. The fault was corrected but, funnily enough, they were no longer so popular and havw subsequently gone out of production.

Medtronic Hall

These have been used since 1977. They have a carbon-coated disc with a unique central hole. The disc is retained and guided by a strut that protrudes through this hole.

Note that acute thrombosis involving mitral valve prostheses can occur and may require urgent thrombolysis to establish enough flow to allow anaesthesia.

Bileaflet valves

St Jude Medical

These were introduced in 1977. They are the most popular valve and have two semi-circulation leaflets, which open and close creating one central and two peripheral lumens.

CarboMedics

These were introduced in 1986. They are like the St Jude Medical model, but with a slightly different hinge mechanism.

Biological valves

Autograft

This involves translocation of a valve within the same individual. In the Ross procedure the native pulmonary valve is moved to the aortic position. The pulmonary valve is replaced by a homograft or a heterograft (see below).

Autologous

This involves making a valve out of the patient's tissue. An example is the Carpentier–Edwards Perimount pericardial prosthesis, which is a frame-mounted valve constructed from the patient's pericardium (in the operating room).

Homograft (allografts)

These are obtained from another human, usually from cadavers, and are stored in fixative or are cryopreserved.

Heterograft (xenografts)

These are obtained from another animal species. They may be mounted on a stent (attached to the sewing ring) or they may be stentless, which offers a greater orifice area.

Examples are:
- Porcine
  - Hancock II porcine (Medtronic Hall)
  - Biocor porcine (St Jude Medical)

- ◦ Carpentier–Edwards supra-annular valve
- Bovine
  - ◦ Carpentier–Edwards pericardial bio-prosthesis (fashioned from bovine pericardium mounted on a stented frame).

PULMONARY VALVE REPLACEMENT

This is increasingly used, especially in long-term Fallot. It is likely that the original pulmonary valves may have been compromised when the right ventricular outflow tract was corrected. Severe pulmonary regurgitation is not uncommon more than 10 years later and can lead to irreversible right ventricular disease. Patients with Fallot are best followed up by the adult congenital heart disease (ACHD) team.

Follow-up

The first follow-up after valve replacement or repair should be 1 month after surgery. This should involve:
- Recording the valve type, name and size
- Bloods for FBC and U&Es
- ECG and chest X-ray
- Echocardiogram (this will be the first postoperative benchmark for future comparison), record:
  - ◦ Function of prosthesis
  - ◦ Gradient (aortic valve) and compare this with the manufacturer's range
  - ◦ Valve area
  - ◦ Chamber dimensions and function
  - ◦ Pulmonary artery pressure from tricuspid regurgitation
  - ◦ Other valvular pathology.

It is good practice to review patients annually for a full history and examination. Order a chest X-ray and echocardiogram only if indicated.

Antibiotic prophylaxis

In high-risk patients, give antibiotics to those with:

- Prosthetic heart valves, including bioprosthetic homograft and allograft valves
- Previous bacterial endocarditis
- Complex cyanotic congenital heart disease (e.g. single ventricle states, transposition of the great arteries, tetralogy of Fallot)
- Surgically constructed systemic-pulmonary shunts or conduits.

In moderate-risk patients, give antibiotics to those with:
- Most other congenital cardiac malformations
- Acquired valvular dysfunction (e.g. rheumatic heart disease)
- Hypertrophic cardiomyopathy with outflow obstruction
- Mitral valve prolapse with auscultatory evidence of valvular regurgitation and/or thickened leaflets.

Check the *British National Formulary* for the most appropriate antibiotic to use. This changes constantly so you should not be expected to remember it.

Anticoagulation

All patients with mechanical prosthetic valves need warfarin and aspirin 75 mg. Patients receiving clopidogrel need not take aspirin.

For the first 3 months all patients need an INR of 2.5–3.5, then for:
- Aortic valves the INR should be 2.0–3.0
- Mitral valves the INR should be 2.5–3.5.

A guide to managing over-anticoagulation is given in **Table 22.**

For anticoagulation for non-cardiac surgery or dental care:
- Stop warfarin 72 hours before the procedure (restart on the day of the procedure if there is no bleeding)
- Admit 48 hours before the procedure and start heparin when the INR is < 2 (APTT: 55–70 seconds)
- Stop heparin 6 hours before the procedure, restart within 24 hours and continue until the INR is > 2.

Table 22. Managing over-anticoagulation	
INR < 7	Withhold warfarin for 24 hours and recheck
INR > 7	Withhold warfarin and give 2.5 mg of vitamin K i.v.
If bleeding: • Life threatening	Give 5 mg of vitamin K i.v. and concentrated clotting factors (or fresh frozen plasma i.v. 1 l if not available)
• Less severe (e.g. epistaxis)	Give 0.5–2.0 mg vitamin K (high-dose or i.v. vitamin K increases the risk of over-correction)

Additional information

Remember:

- Mechanical valves do not have vegetations on them when they become infected
- Haemolysis is not uncommon with mechanical valves, but it is usually mild and well tolerated. However, if it is more severe suspect a para-prosthetic leak
- Always ask for an echocardiogram if a patient with a prosthetic valve is failing to thrive or if they are due for an operation
- Remember that a xenograft will normally last around 10–15 years.

Cardiomyopathies

Nick Fisher

DILATED CARDIOMYOPATHY

You need to tackle this condition by serial elimination of aetiologies, and you will probably end up with a diagnosis of idiopathic dilated cardiomyopathy (IDC). IDC is treated in a similar way to chronic heart failure, so that's easy. However, before you pat yourself on the back and reach for the ACE inhibitors, make really sure that you have not missed a reversible (non-idiopathic) cause or previously missed systemic disease.

Presentation

Patients present the same way as do patients with left ventricular failure. However, not infrequently they are picked up at routine medicals or when screening for familial disease.

History

Ask about:
- History consistent with ischaemic heart disease
- Recent illnesses with a possible viral cause
- Family history of heart failure or premature death
- Blood disorders, such as thalassaemia and haemochromatosis
- Risk factors for HIV
- Alcohol intake (how much *precisely*)
- Cocaine use
- Systemic, connective tissue type problems.

Investigations

Blood tests

You should order the following blood tests:

- FBC
- U&Es
- Liver function tests (note: gamma-glutamyltransferase in big drinkers)
- Thyroid function tests
- Iron studies (thalassaemia, haemochromatosis)
- Creatinine kinase (muscular dystrophy)
- Viral titres (in adults the relation between viral titres and chronic IDC is uncertain, so detecting viral antibodies adds little to the management).

When appropriate, consider:

- Autoantibodies
- Carnitine
- Lactate/pyruvate
- Selenium
- Acyl carnitine profile
- Drug screen
- Red cell transketolase (beriberi)
- Infective screen (HIV, hepatitis C, enteroviruses).

Electrocardiography

The ECG is usually remarkably normal. Remember supraventricular tachycardia and ventricular tachycardia is more frequent, and any suggestions of palpitations or syncope should trigger you to order a 24-hour tape.

Echocardiography

It will come as no surprise that you are looking for a dilated left ventricle. However, a useful criterion for a dilated cardiomyopathy is a left ventricular dimension > 112% predicted normal value. Abnormal systolic function can also be defined as an ejection fraction of < 45% or a shortening fraction of < 25%.

Cardiac MRI

The ability of cardiac MRI to determine chamber size, function and volume and cardiac mass is little more than an echocardiogram could achieve. However, if available, late gadolinium uptake images can be invaluable for establishing an ischaemic (silent infarct) picture.

Nuclear perfusion

Request nuclear perfusion if the history indicates that the patient may have an ischaemic element, and the patient is unsuitable for an exercise tolerance test. Obviously, move on to angiography if there is significant reversible ischaemia.

Urine

Test for vanillylmandelic acid levels. A result twice that of normal is often diagnostic for phaeochromocytoma. One collection should be enough. Refer patients with an elevated level to an endocrinologist, who will probably organise plasma noradrenaline. Remember that a phaeochromocytoma can cause a cardiomyopathy so severe that the blood pressure may be normal.

HYPERTROPHIC CARDIOMYOPATHY

Hypertrophic cardiomyopathy (HCM) is a diagnosis that covers a broad spectrum of disease, and to describe someone as having the condition confers about as much information as saying they have a brown car.

The approach to managing a patient with this condition is:
- Accurate diagnosis
- Accurate history
- Treatment of symptoms
- Risk stratification.

Risk stratification is most important because some patients are at a much higher risk of sudden cardiac death than others.

Investigations
History
Ask about:
- Exertional dyspnoea
- Impaired consciousness
- Chest pain
- Syncope
- Palpitations
- Family history of HCM, arrhythmias, syncope or premature death.

Electrocardiography
The ECG is often abnormal, from left ventricular hypertrophy to gross repolarisation abnormalities. These offer no prognostic information. Note that a slurred upstroke to a broad QRS complex is not that unusual, but an accessory pathway is found in less than 5% of patients.

With deep inverted T waves think of apical HCM, and don't be misled by a normal echocardiograph – ask for a cardiac MRI.

Echocardiography
The classic pattern is:
- Asymmetrical septal hypertrophy
- Systolic anterior motion of the mitral valve
- Dynamic left ventricular outflow tract obstruction.

Record maximal myocardial thickness (in diastole), anatomical location and outflow tract gradient. Remember that it is extremely difficult to pick up apical HCM with an echocardiogram.

Holter monitoring
Up to 30% of patients will have non-sustained supraventricular tachycardia. More sinister is non-sustained ventricular tachycardia, which up to 20% of patients will have. The absence of non-sustained ventricular tachycardia is a good negative predictor.

Exercise-tolerance testing

Look for an abnormal blood-pressure response to exercise testing. This is defined as a failure to augment and/or sustain a systolic blood pressure of > 25 mmHg that of resting blood pressure during exercise.

You will see it in about 25% of patients, making its positive predictive value for sudden cardiac death low. It is more sensitive in patients who are younger than 40 years.

Genetic testing

Obviously, some mutations in HCM carry prognostic significance. However, this is far from straightforward because the genotype–phenotype relationship has not been fully clarified. Currently, testing should be left to specialist centres.

Cardiac MRI

Cardiac MRI offers two main advantages over echocardiography in patients with HCM. First, the ventricular morphology can be beautifully determined. This is particularly important with suspected apical HCM (unexplained inverted T waves) because gross apical abnormalities can be missed with echocardiography in these patients.

Second, a new finding is that uptake of late gadolinium (which can be grossly abnormal in HCM) correlates well with high-risk patients. This is currently being validated.

Sudden cardiac death

A risk assessment for sudden cardiac death is given in **Table 23**. Offer the patient an implantable cardioverter defibrillator (ICD) as prophylaxis against sudden death in patients:

- With two or more of the risk factors listed in Table 23 (and/or amiodarone)
- Who have had a cardiac arrest or who have sustained or symptomatic ventricular tachycardia.

Table 23. Risk assessment for sudden cardiac death

Give one point for each positive:

History	• Syncope (especially exertional) • Family history of sudden cardiac death • Previous cardiac arrest
Echocardiogram	• Severe (≥ 3 cm of hypertrophy)
Holter monitoring	• Non-sustained ventricular tachycardia
Exercise-tolerance test	• Abnormal blood-pressure response

Remember, more than 60% of sudden cardiac deaths occur during or immediately after exercise. Patients should at least avoid strenuous or competitive sports.

Treatment
Outflow tract obstruction
Medical treatment consists of:
- Beta blockers (atenolol 50–100 mg od)
- +/– disopyramide 150–400 mg bd.

Disopyramide can be added to beta blockers, but should not be used instead of beta blockers because they can accelerate AV conduction (this is not good if the patient develops a supraventricular tachycardia). Disopyramide can help reduce symptoms and outflow gradient. High doses are often needed, but side effects may become an issue.

Verapamil may cause possible peripheral vasodilatation and haemodynamic collapse; it is best to avoid these drugs in patients with obstruction.

If the resting outflow gradient is > 50 mmHg and medical treatment is not effective, consider removing the outflow obstruction by:

- Myomectomy – this has a success rate of 80% with maintained relief in 70%. Mortality is 2%.
- Alcohol septal ablation – alcohol is injected into the septal perforators of the left anterior descending artery to cause a limited myocardial infarction.

Pacing was in vogue a few years ago, but there was a significant placebo effect. This is not now used very often.

No outflow tract obstruction

Treatment is as follows:

- Beta blocker (atenolol 50–100 mg od)
- Calcium antagonist (verapamil 80–160 mg tds; diltiazem 300–400 mg od).

If dilatation and systolic function deteriorate, add ACE inhibitors etc. as for chronic heart failure.

Arrhythmias

- Treat as these as normal – you can safely use amiodarone
- Some 30% of patients have a supraventricular tachycardia
- A slurred upstroke to a broad QRS complex is a normal variant
- An accessory pathway can be found in < 5% of patients.

Pacemakers

Nick Fisher
Jeff Davison
Richard Sutton

PACEMAKER NOMENCLATURE AND TYPES

Pacemaker nomenclature is given in **Table 24**. Common types of pacemakers are given in **Table 25**.

Table 24. Pacemaker nomenclature

Pacemakers are described with a three-letter code. Sometimes there may be a fourth letter (see below)

Letter 1	Describes where stimulation occurs	• A (atrium) • V (ventricle) • D (dual – both atrium and ventricle)
Letter 2	Describes where sensing occurs	• A (atrium) • V (ventricle) • D (dual – both atrium and ventricle)
Letter 3	Describes the mode of sensing	• I (a sensed event inhibits) • T (an output pulse is triggered by a sensed event) • D (dual – both T and I can occur [only on dual chamber devices])

In some models a fourth letter (R) will be added to indicate rate modulation. These pacemakers will detect patient movement and speed up accordingly in an attempt to recreate a physiological response.

Table 25. Common types of pacemaker

AAI (plus R if chronotropic incompetence)	For people with sinus node diseases and normal AV conduction
VVI (plus R if chronotropic incompetence)	For people with chronic atrial fibrillation with no hope of being in sinus rhythm. These are sometimes used for cost reasons in very elderly patients with co-morbid conditions and little ambulation
DDD (plus R if chronotropic incompetence)	Most other pacemakers are of this type

INDICATIONS FOR PERMANENT PACEMAKER IMPLANTATION

Indications for a permanent pacemaker implant are:

- Complete heart block, even if asymptomatic
- Type II heart block
  - Mobitz 1 (Wenckebach), when symptomatic only
  - Mobitz 2, even if asymptomatic
- Bifascicular/trifascicular block – if you are unable to establish a non-cardiac cause for syncope then assume it is due to transient complete heart block and pace. However, efforts to establish the cause of syncope are mandatory. Remember that neurally mediated syncope and ventricular tachycardia is a lot more common than AV block
- Sinus node dysfunction (sick sinus syndrome) – you need documented symptomatic bradycardia (in some patients this may be due to unavoidable medication)
- Atrial fibrillation with symptomatic pauses of > 3 seconds
- Hypertensive carotid sinus syndrome – this is not very common, but increasingly recognised. When the correct diagnostic protocol is followed it is a firm indication for pacing. You

need to demonstrate syncope associated with carotid sinus massage (CSM) where minimal carotid sinus pressure induces asystole of > 3 seconds.

Note that CSM should be performed supine and erect using equipment capable of beat-to-beat monitoring of the ECG complexes.

New indications
Heart failure
Biventricular pacing is now becoming more popular. Left ventricle pacing is best achieved by a coronary sinus lead; there is evidence of benefit in patients with severe congestive heart failure (NYHA class III or IV) and left bundle branch block with a broad QRS > 120 ms.

Hypertrophic cardiomyopathy
It may be beneficial to dual chamber pace patients with symptomatic outflow tract obstruction. This is done by pacing patients with a short AV delay from the right ventricular apex, resulting in a paradoxical septal motion that reduces outflow obstruction. However, the success of catheter septal ablation has led to the decline of this procedure.

Vasovagal syncope
In patients who have documented syncopal episodes during head-up tilt-table testing with associated bradycardia, a pacemaker can be effective.

You need a rate-drop response unit that detects sudden bradycardic episodes and increases the heart rate above and beyond normal. This will compensate for the hypotension that is caused not only by bradycardia, but peripheral vasodilatation associated with increased vagal tone. This is called a flywheel effect.

PRE-OPERATIVE CARE
On the day of the pacemaker implantation follow the steps described below.

Consent

Quote the following risks:

- Bruising: 20%
- Haematoma: 5%
- Lead repositioning: 7%
- Pneumothorax: 1%
- Pericardial effusion: 1%.

Prophylactic antibiotics

Give co–amoxiclav (Augmentin) 625 mg tds for 3 days. (Gentamicin 80 mg should also be given into the pocket during the procedure.)

Document

You should *clearly* document:

- INR (needs to be < 1.5)
- Haemoglobin
- Platelets
- Urea
- Creatinine
- Potassium.

Venflon

This should be inserted on the side of the implant because it allows contrast media to be injected if the subclavian vein is hard to find.

ADDITIONAL INFORMATION

Remember:

- Pacemakers are fitted into the non-dominant side so that they are less likely to move during activity
- A and V leads are inserted into the right atrium and right ventricle via the subclavian or cephalic veins
- Patients with previous cardiac surgery have often lost their atrial appendage because it is opened to aid cardiac bypass during the procedure. Normally, atrial leads are positioned in

the appendage for stability, so a fixation lead (which has a small corkscrew that winds into the endocardium) is usually used to enable a stable position elsewhere. The injury caused by the fixation often leads to a higher stimulation threshold, which will fall with time

- Departments often deliberately use a mixture of boxes and leads supplied by different manufacturers. This is a damage-limitation exercise in case of a product recall that could potentially involve all your patients.

PACEMAKER VALUES

At the time of positioning, correct placement is confirmed by obtaining the values given in **Table 26**.

Once these values have been confirmed the patient is paced at a maximum voltage of 10 V in the A and V leads, and the operator's hand is placed on the abdomen to check there is no diaphragmatic capture (which will cause twitching or hiccups).

Table 26. Pacemaker values		
A lead Intrinsic ECG for injury potential (confirms a good contact and excludes perforation)	• **A-wave amplitude** (how well it will sense)	2–3 mV
	• **Threshold** (minimum voltage required to get capture)	< 1 V at 0.5 ms
	• **Slew** (the change in voltage and reflecting ability to sense)	> 0.3 V/s
V lead Intrinsic ECG for injury potential	• **V wave**	> 6 mV
	• **Threshold**	< 1 V
	• **Slew**	> 0.5 V/s

POST-OPERATIVE CARE

Post-operative care should involve:

- Ordering a chest X-ray to document (and check) the lead position (**Figure 3**) and to check for pneumothorax if subclavian puncture was used
- Checking the closure material used (most people use subcutaneous Dexon, which dissolves on its own)
- Checking the pacemaker – usually carried out by a technician to ensure that the values have remained stable (often the thresholds and impedance increase slightly, reflecting underlying oedema at the lead tips). Any fancy programming of the device will occur at this stage.

Patient advice

Advise patients:

- Don't raise their arm on the side of unit above their shoulder for 1 week
- Keep the wound dry for 1 week

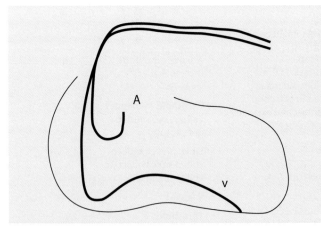

Figure 3. Typical lead positions showing the amount of 'slack' you would expect to see in each lead.

- Don't drive for 1 week
- Hold mobile phones to the opposite ear. Do not keep mobile phones in a pocket overlying the generator
- They may undergo computed tomography (CT) scans but **NOT** MRI scans
- Pacemakers need to be checked after cardioversion and radio-therapy
- Prophylactic antibiotics are **NOT** needed for dental work
- To inform airport checkpoints that they have a pacemaker and to produce the card given to them by the technician
- Microwaves are safe
- Avoid working on car-ignition systems, high-tension electrical power sources and arc welding systems
- Avoid contact sports (also avoid using a rifle with the stock against the pacemaker).

COMMON POST-PROCEDURE COMPLICATIONS
Pneumothorax

This is seen when a subclavian vein is used and there was difficulty gaining access. Treat as any pneumothorax (i.e. don't go diving in with a chest drain unless really necessary).

Lead displacement

This may be obvious from the chest X-ray. If there are markedly raised thresholds and impedance it needs repositioning with a fixation lead. If within 3 months there are no significant radiographic changes and there is a moderate increase in thresholds and impedance, give the patient a week's worth of reducing prednisolone (30 mg, 20 mg, 10 mg, 5mg: 2 days each).

Haematoma

These can be quite large. Understandably many doctors are tempted to evacuate them, but you risk infection if you do this. Avoid this unless bleeding continues, the sutures are coming apart, skin is breaking down or the pain is uncontrolled by analgesics. **DO NOT** aspirate the haematoma.

Ventricular perforation

This is often indicated during lead placement by an intracardiac ECG that looks remarkably like a surface one! This is not uncommon; the lead is simply gently withdrawn and placed elsewhere. However, you should document this and book an echocardiogram later that day to ensure that a significant pericardial effusion has not occurred. This is unlikely, but potentially serious. Treat as any effusion.

Later complications

Pacemaker syndrome

Pacemaker syndrome is less common now that we use dual chamber devices in nearly all patients. However, it is important to recognise it in patients with VVI devices who are suitable for an upgrade. It consists of light-headedness or syncope and sometimes episodic weakness. It is related to long periods of AV asynchrony or 1:1 retrograde AV conduction occurring during ventricular-inhibited pacing.

Lead dislodgement

Treat as described above.

Lead fracture

This occurs at stress points, usually where the leads pass under the clavicle, or due to direct trauma. As a short-term solution bipolar systems can usually be programmed as unipolar to resume pacing. Analysis of the lead will indicate increased impedance in these cases. If there is a break in the insulation the impedance will be low. However, if there is a lead fracture with the conductor only breaking, the impedance will be high.

Twiddler syndrome

Some people just can't resist a fiddle with their box and have an amazing ability to coil their leads up. If you see an unbelievable lead pattern or box position this could be the problem.

Infection

This usually presents as a localised pocket infection. Expert senior help is needed because treatment usually involves removing the whole system, which is easier said than done. Leads become incorporated into the endothelium of vessels and the endocardial surface with time, and specialised extraction techniques as well as a good tug are often needed.

Erosion

Erosion is due to inadequate depth of placement or possible infection. Impending erosion should be treated as an emergency because if the skin is perforated the whole system will most likely need to be replaced.

Skin tethering

This is due to inadequate depth of placement and more often occurs in thin people. If the skin is viable and healthy it should be watched more frequently, but if there is danger of the skin breaking down then the pocket will need to be revised.

PACED ECG PROBLEMS
Tip extrasystoles

In the first day or so after pacemaker insertion you can sometimes see ventricular complexes that appear without a preceding pacing spike, but that look the same as the paced complexes. They are 'tip extrasystoles' and usually resolve spontaneously.

Failure to capture

Here, pacing is seen with no subsequent QRS complex. A technician needs to check this.

Failure to pace

With this problem, pauses will occur where you would expect to see a paced beat. This can be due to any inherent fault with the box or lead. It can also be due to the system oversensing. With a dual-chamber system there may be A activity without subsequent V activity. This is often caused by the atrial activity being over sensed by the V lead (cross talk). A technician needs to check this.

Failure to sense
Here, you will see inappropriate spikes following intrinsic cardiac activity. This is often due to dislodgement. A technician needs to check this.

Rate is too slow
Are you sure? Many pacemakers have a programmed hysteresis rate that is lower than the pacemaker base rate. If the patient's rate falls below the hysteresis rate, the pacemaker cuts in at its faster base rate. If in doubt, place a magnet over the box and it will default to a set-pacing rate of 60–80 bpm.

Pulse is irregular
If the pulse is irregular, check the ECG. The pacemaker may well be appropriately sensing/pacing with varying cardiac outputs.

Common cardiac arrhythmias and implantable cardioverter defibrillators

Nick Fisher
Bilal Iqbal
Malcolm Finlay

INTRODUCTION

This chapter is in line with guidelines from the American College of Cardiology, the American Heart Association and the European Society of Cardiology.[2,8,9]

First, here are some things that we pretend to know but often forget!

- Heart rate = 300/RR interval (measured in big squares)
- Rhythm is either regular or irregularly irregular (atrial fibrillation and Wenckebach are the only truly irregular rhythms)
- Each little square is 40 ms
- Normal PR interval (measured from the **start** of the P wave to the **start** of the QRS) = 120–200 ms
- A PR interval longer than this indicates first-degree AV block
- A progressively lengthening PR interval indicates second-degree AV block (Mobitz I; Wenckebach)
- A constant PR with missed beats indicates second-degree AV block (Mobitz II)
- Complete PR dissociation indicates third-degree AV block or complete heart block
- Normal QRS is < 120 ms

- QT (measured from the **start** of the QRS to the **end** of the T wave) – correct for rate (QT_c) to 60 beats/min by using equation $QT_c = (QT)/(\sqrt{RR})$ where RR is the RR interval. All times in **seconds**. Normal is 0.35–0.43 s
- Axis – as a rule of thumb, look at the predominant deflection in leads I, II and III. Note how II and III move as one.

BASIC COMMON SENSE

The diagnosis and treatment of arrhythmias seem to provoke fear in many of us. However, shielded by a cloak of mystique lie some basic principles that will allow you to easily deal with most cases. Remember that common things are common, and despite the list of potential diagnoses there are few that we see 99% of the time.

Remember, tachycardias can be divided into broad or narrow complex tachycardias.

Broad complex tachycardias

With broad complex tachycardias the QRS is >120 ms. They include:

- Supraventricular tachycardia with bundle branch block or aberrant conduction
- Supraventricular tachycardia conducted through an accessory pathway
- Ventricular tachycardia.

There is no reliable rule that will distinguish these. Patients with a broad complex tachycardia that are in anyway compromised should be treated as for ventricular tachycardia by the advanced life support guidelines. If the patient is well, see management of ventricular tachycardia below.

Narrow complex tachycardias

With narrow complex tachycardias the QRS is < 120 ms. Remember:

- Patients with atrial fibrillation have an irregularly irregular rhythm and no P waves

- Pre-excitation (see below) on the 12-lead ECG and symptomatic tachycardias indicate Wolff–Parkinson–White syndrome
- A regular rhythm with a rate of 150 ms is very likely to be flutter (with 2:1 block). Look for P waves hidden at a rate of 300 ms
- Other regular tachycardias are most likely to be AV nodal re-entrant tachycardias. They look like flutter but are often faster and there are no P waves.

Adenosine

If vagal manoeuvres (e.g. CSM) do not terminate an acute supraventricular tachycardia then give adenosine. Classically, you start at 3 mg i.v. and titrate up in 3 mg stages. However, you might as well give a good 12 mg dose and be sure to treat the problem. Some 90% of re-entrant tachycardias will be terminated by this dose. It will also help you exclude supraventricular tachycardia in broad complex tachycardias.

Remember:
- Warn patients that they will feel flushed and short of breath or 'queer', with chest tightness, but this will last less than 20 seconds
- Be careful in patients with asthma with significant disease (we wouldn't give adenosine if they have ever been admitted to the intensive care unit for acute asthma)
- Heart transplant patients are becoming more common and are very sensitive to adenosine
- Don't give adenosine to patients with atrial fibrillation. It won't convert the rhythm and if they have an accessory pathway it may encourage its use in preference to the AV node, increasing the rate and inducing ventricular fibrillation!

NEW-ONSET ATRIAL FIBRILLATION IN THE CLINIC
Diagnosis

Diagnosis requires an ECG. This sounds obvious, but referrals of patients with an irregular pulse and a clinical diagnosis of atrial fibrillation are common. If the R-R interval is irregularly irregular then it is atrial fibrillation (Wenckebach is the exception, but this has regular P waves).

Confirm the diagnosis by:
* Looking at an ECG!
* If the patient is in sinus rhythm when you see them and there is no ECG from the referring doctor, consider paroxysmal atrial fibrillation (order a 24-hour ECG) and request a copy of the ECG from the referring doctor.

Next, consider the aetiology. Although atrial fibrillation can occur as part of normal ageing without an obvious precipitating cause, this is only a diagnosis of exclusion.

History
Ask about:
* Binge drinking or excessive drinking (holiday heart syndrome)
* Smoking or symptoms of ischaemic heart disease
* Drug misuse
* Infections
* Weight loss (cancer, hyperthyroidism).

Examination
Look for:
* Goitre/exophthalmos
* Lung effusion/consolidation
* Hypertension
* Murmurs (especially mitral valve disease).

Investigations
Order the following:
* Bloods
  * U&Es
  * Magnesium

- ○ Thyroid function tests
- ○ Lipids
- ○ Glucose
- ○ Liver function tests (with gamma-glutamyltransferase)
- Chest X-ray (don't forget to look at the lungs as well as the heart
- Echocardiogram
  - ○ Left atrial size (> 5 cm, less likely to stay in sinus rhythm)
  - ○ Ventricular dimensions and function
  - ○ Valve pathology (especially mitral valve).

Treatment

The treatment of atrial fibrillation obviously depends on aetiology, age and co-existent pathology. Wherever possible, your aims should be to restore sinus rhythm and then to maintain it. Failing this, you should aim for adequate anticoagulation and rate control.

The general treatment of atrial fibrillation consists of two main components:

- Management of arrhythmia
  - ○ Drugs for rate control/rhythm control (see below)
- Anticoagulation
  - ○ Warfarin/aspirin (see below).

Many algorithms have been produced to guide us through the treatment of new-onset atrial fibrillation. The patient-based examples in **Tables 27–29** should help you to make some sense of them.

Note that warfarin (where the patient has not had heparin) is pro-coagulant. Therefore, consider giving concomitant heparin if the risk of thrombus formation is high (large left atrium, very poor left ventricle, etc).

Table 27. The patient with reversible pathology*

1. Treat the precipitating cause
2. Anticoagulate: give warfarin (INR 2–3)
3. Control rate: digoxin/beta blocker/calcium antagonist (depending on left ventricular function)
4. Aim to cardiovert when the precipitating cause has been removed
5. If sinus rhythm is established continue warfarin until follow-up. Check in 4 weeks to establish sinus rhythm, but stop digoxin/beta blocker/calcium antagonist

* Hyperthyroidism, pneumonia, alcohol binge, etc.

Table 28. The patient with no obvious precipitating cause

1. Anticoagulate: give warfarin (INR 2–3)
2. Control rate: digoxin/beta blocker/calcium antagonist (depending on left ventricular function)
3. Aim to cardiovert after 6 weeks of appropriate anticoagulation
4. If sinus rhythm is established, continue warfarin until follow-up. Check in 4 weeks to establish sinus rhythm, but stop digoxin/beta blocker/calcium antagonist

Amiodarone

Remember:

- Amiodarone dosage is 200 mg tds 1/52, 200 mg bd 1/52 and 200 mg od maintenance
- Amiodarone potentiates warfarin and can significantly increase the INR (see Chapter 14).
- Inform patients and their GP of the need for thyroid function tests (it is a good idea to have baseline thyroid function tests before you start)
- Inform the patient of the effects of sun and corneal deposits on their vision
- A 100 mg dose is a useful compromise between side effects and long-term prophylaxis.

> **Table 29. The patient with other pathology likely to precipitate repeated atrial fibrillation**
>
> These are typically patients with heart failure, ischaemic heart disease or mitral valve disease that may not be severe enough to warrant surgery. The left ventricular dysfunction, with or without mitral regurgitation, causes atrial dilatation and strain, and makes atrial fibrillation much more likely. These patients will often have a lot to gain from sinus rhythm, and they should be offered the chance of cardioversion. Remember, atrial contractions can contribute up to 20% of the cardiac output.
>
> 1. Anticoagulate: give warfarin (INR 2–3)
> 2. Control rate:
>   - If there is hypertension or ischaemic heart disease use a beta blocker (atenolol or sotalol)
>   - If there is heart failure, use digoxin or amiodarone
>   - In very resistant atrial fibrillation, use amiodarone
> 3. Aim to cardiovert after 6 weeks of appropriate anticoagulation, but continue the beta blocker or amiodarone to maintain sinus rhythm
> 4. Follow up with a 24-hour tape if paroxysmal atrial fibrillation is likely and review in the clinic 1 month later
> 5. If sinus rhythm has been maintained, stop the warfarin. Patients with paroxysmal atrial fibrillation with thromboembolic risk factors warrant long-term anticoagulation with warfarin (see algorithm below)

Anticoagulation

Remember:

- Patients with atrial fibrillation have a six-fold increased risk of stroke. Consider anticoagulation in **ALL** patients, regardless of the pattern of the arrhythmia
- Elderly patients are often denied anticoagulation because of a presumed increased risk of haemorrhagic complications. For these patients with a high thrombo-embolic risk, current trial data suggest the benefits of anticoagulation may be greater (if there are no contraindications)

- For stable patients, in whom the onset of atrial fibrillation is uncertain or longer than 48 hours, anticoagulation for a minimum of 3 weeks is recommended before cardioversion to allow resolution of potential thrombi. Because atrial mechanical activity may not resume concurrently with electrical activity, anticoagulation should be continued for at least four weeks after cardioversion
- Be aware of the potential drug interactions of warfarin (see Chapter 14).

Which antithrombotic agent should you use? Remember, anticoagulation therapy needs to be tailored to the individual patient, based on age, co-morbidities and contraindications. Patients can be stratified into high, intermediate and low risk for stroke (**Figure 4**).

Cardioversion

The patient will usually come in as a day case, usually first thing. You will need:
- An anaesthetist
- A cardiac defibrillator
- An INR > 2 (documented as being consistently above 2 for 6 weeks)
- Nursing staff
- A signed consent form (quote the risks of stroke [~1%] and burns on the chest. Also warn the patient that cardioversion might not work)
- Current ECG showing the patient is still in atrial fibrillation.

Once the patient is asleep, turn on the monitor strip record, SYNC the defibrillator, and defibrillate with 200 J DC (50 J biphasic) shock, followed by 360 J (100 J biphasic) if unsuccessful. Don't rush. If you are uncertain whether defibrillation was successful, print off a rhythm strip and ask "Is it regular?"

In patients in whom ventricular standstill is a real concern, ensure the defibrillator also has transcutaneous pacing facilities. If in doubt, always use such a defibrillator.

RHYTHM OR RATE CONTROL

Recent trials have cast doubt on the necessity of maintaining sinus rhythm, compared with anticoagulation and rate control. We think these trials confirm that it is perfectly safe to treat asympto-

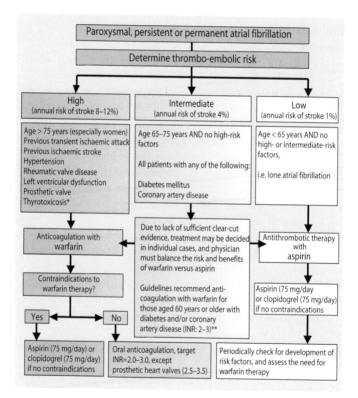

Figure 4. Algorithm for anticoagulating patients with atrial fibrillation. Reproduced from *BMJ* 2005;330:238–243 with permission from the BMJ Publishing Group.

* Thyrotoxicosis is associated with a high thrombo-embolic risk in atrial fibrillation. Current guidelines recommend anticoagulation with warfarin, if no contraindications exist, at least until a euthyroid state is achieved and congestive heart failure has been corrected. ** Patients with coronary artery disease may have additional therapy with low-dose aspirin (75 mg/day) or low-dose clopidogrel (75 mg/day). This has not been evaluated sufficiently and may be associated with increased risk of bleeding.

matic patients who are unlikely to remain in sinus rhythm or in whom cardioversion has been unsuccessful and who are often elderly with rate control. It does not mean that younger or symptomatic patients, especially those with structurally normal hearts, should not be returned to sinus rhythm.

Rhythm control
Remember:
- Identify and treat all reversible causes of atrial fibrillation before considering drug therapy for maintenance of sinus rhythm
- Tailor your choice of anti-arrhythmic drug to the patient, depending on cardiac status, co-morbidities and contraindications
- In patients with good left ventricular function and no coronary artery disease, flecainide and propafenone can be used. You can also use sotalol or amiodarone in these patients
- Amiodarone can be used to maintain sinus rhythm in patients with heart failure
- Consider sotalol for patients with coronary artery disease (it has class III and beta-blocking effects)
- If sinus rhythm cannot be maintained, despite repeated cardioversions and anti-arrhythmic therapy, adopt a rate-control strategy. This has been shown to be equally as effective
- Patients who find the symptoms of the arrhythmia unacceptable despite rate control may be considered for non-pharmacological methods to restore sinus rhythm.

Rate control
Remember:
- Digoxin is ineffective for controlling ventricular rate during acute episodes and paroxysmal episodes, and in states with high sympathetic tone such as thyrotoxicosis and critical illness, and in postoperative states
- In patients with good left ventricular function, beta blockers (metoprolol, atenolol and sotalol) or non-dihydropyridine calcium antagonists (verapamil and diltiazem) are the drugs of choice, provided there are no contraindications

- In patients with acute or chronic heart failure, digoxin or amiodarone should be used. Chronic use of amiodarone is limited by its side effects. Consider beta blockers in patients with stable heart failure
- Although digoxin does not provide good rate control in acute episodes, it is generally effective for rate control in persistent atrial fibrillation
- Consider combination therapy when adequate rate control cannot be achieved with a single drug. A combination of digoxin and atenolol or diltiazem is effective
- Assess the adequacy of rate control by the clinical symptoms
- Target heart rates vary with age. They should generally be 60–90 bpm at rest and 90–115 bpm during exercise. This requires careful dose titration
- Poor ventricular rate control in the long term leads to a reversible deterioration of left ventricular function (tachycardiomyopathy).

PAROXYSMAL ATRIAL FIBRILLATION

Management of paroxysmal atrial fibrillation in the clinic is not very different from that of persistent/permanent atrial fibrillation. However, because the patient is in and out of sinus rhythm anyway, you don't need to cardiovert them, just to stabilise them in sinus rhythm.

First, confirm they are having paroxysms of atrial fibrillation with a 24-hour tape. Remember that palpitations can be caused by atrioventricular node re-entry tachycardias (AVRTs), ventricular tachycardia, flutter, sinus tachycardia and heart block, as well as psychogenic causes. The risk of stroke in paroxysmal atrial fibrillation remains and is obviously related to the duration and extent of paroxysms and presence of co-morbid risk factors. You should therefore have a low threshold for anticoagulation.

Once again, if the patient has hypertension or ischaemic heart disease use atenolol (25–50 mg od) or sotalol (40–80mg bd). With its additional class III activity, sotalol is probably better if there is no obvious indication for atenolol.

In young people with no structural or ischaemic heart disease, flecainide (50–100 mg bd) avoids the side effects of beta blockers and is just as effective.

POST-OPERATIVE ATRIAL TACHYCARDIAS

Pericardial inflammation, catecholamines and autonomic dysfunction all make atrial arrhythmias more likely after cardiac surgery. You should remember the following points in addition to those above. The most common cause of atrial fibrillation post-operatively is, however, either volume overload or an underloaded heart, especially where volume changes are sudden.

- Patients receiving beta blockers pre-operatively should continue to receive them.
- Thrombogenicity is enhanced and anticoagulation should be started for any supraventricular tachycardia (permanent or paroxysmal) occurring after 24 hours.
- The efficacy of digoxin will be reduced by catecholamines and may require higher doses.
- The arrhythmias are often transient, therefore ensure cardiological review at 6–8 weeks to consider withdrawal of anticoagulation and to review medication.

ATRIOVENTRICULAR RECIPROCAL TACHYCARDIAS/WOLFF–PARKINSON–WHITE SYNDROME

Tissue connecting the atria and the ventricles, capable of conducting electricity and separate from the AV node, is called an accessory pathway. If it conducts from an atrium to a ventricle it is 'manifest', i.e. it reveals itself on the 12-lead ECG as pre-excitation (the delta wave). Wolff–Parkinson–White syndrome is the combination of pre-excitation *and* symptomatic tachycardias.

Most of these tachycardias are atrioventricular reciprocating tachycardias, which are mediated cyclical circuits passing through the AV node and accessory pathway.

Sudden death

The other less common arrhythmia in Wolff–Parkinson–White syndrome is atrial fibrillation, which if conducted down the accessory pathway can cause rapid ventricular rates, ventricular fibrillation and death. The risk of this is relatively low (< 0.4% over a 10-year follow-up), but it is worth noting that for at least 50% of these patients presenting with a ventricular fibrillation arrest it will be the first time the diagnosis is made. Therefore, the success and relative safety of accessory pathway ablation means that you should consider it in all patients with the condition.

Diagnosis

12-lead ECG

This will show pre-excitation, i.e. early depolarisation (delta wave) of the ventricle down the abnormal pathway. You can tell where the pathway is by going back to first principles. The delta wave will be positive if it is depolarising *towards* that ECG lead:

- If the accessory pathway is depolarising down the right ventricle (anterior pathway), the left ventricle will depolarise late, so the delta wave will begin to resemble a left bundle branch block pattern
- If the accessory pathway is depolarising down the left ventricle (posterior pathway), the left ventricle will depolarise early so the delta wave will begin to resemble a right bundle branch block pattern.

It sounds complex, but if you draw it out you'll be able to nonchalantly impress your colleagues.

24-hour tape

This will demonstrate runs of tachycardia or abnormal conduction (if this occurs while recording). Most importantly, it will differentiate between atrial fibrillation and other supraventricular tachycardias.

Treatment

Electrophysiological testing and accessory pathway ablation

This is a day-case procedure. The ventricle, atrium and normal and abnormal pathways are 'looked at' by internal electrodes inserted via the femoral vein. It is low risk, but bruising in the groin is a possibility. The main serious complications are stroke (< 1%) and complete heart block requiring a pacemaker (~1%). The procedure is done under sedation or a general anaesthetic.

Drugs

As mentioned above, ablation should be the first treatment choice. If the patient is unwilling to be considered for this then flecainide or sotalol are suitable alternatives.

ATRIOVENTRICULAR NODE RE-ENTRY TACHYCARDIAS

Atrioventricular nodal reciprocating tachycardia describes a tachycardia mediated by a re-entrant circuit in the AV node causing the clinical symptom of palpitations. The re-entrant tachycardia circuit is not confined to the AV node; a more modern viewpoint recognises the participation of atrial conduction tissue lying next to the node in the re-entrant circuit.

Electrophysiological data in humans show the fast pathway to be usually located near the apex of Koch's triangle and the slow pathway to extend infero-posteriorly to the AV node along the septal margin of the tricuspid annulus at the level of the coronary sinus. After conduction through the slow pathway to the bundle of His, and therefore transmission to the ventricles, the impulse is transmitted back up the fast pathway to the atria, resulting in a P wave very close to the QRS complex, often obscured by the T wave of the preceding beat.

Diagnosis

Symptoms are:

- Paroxysmal palpitations

- Associated dizziness
- Pulsations in the neck veins, due to the contraction of the atria against the closed tricuspid valve.

Increased atrial pressures also cause release of atrial natriuretic peptide. Paroxysms can therefore be associated with polyuria.

The 12-lead ECG will show characteristic changes. The rapid transmission of the impulse back to the atria results in a P wave rapidly following or obscured by the QRS complex. This results in the pathognomonic ECG changes of a pseudo R wave in V1 and accentuated S waves in 2, 3 and a ventricular fibrillation with a narrow complex tachycardia. Following conversion to sinus rhythm the ECG becomes normal.

You should also order a 24-hour tape.

Treatment
The decision to treat depends, as always, on the exact clinical scenario you are faced with.

Catheter ablation
Definitive treatment is ablation of the slow pathway along the postero-septal region of the tricuspid annulus. This should be offered as a potential cure to all patients with troublesome atrioventricular re-entry tachycardias.

Drugs
These can be used as long-term prophylaxis.
- Verapamil (480 mg in divided doses) is the first-line therapy
- Other choices include class 1 drugs (flecainide, propafenone) and class 3 drugs (amiodarone, sotalol)
- 'The pill in the pocket' – for patients with occasional well-tolerated (but irritating) paroxysms of atrioventricular node re-entry tachycardias who do not wish to undergo catheter ablation or be on long-term pharmacoprophylaxis, you can offer a dose of oral flecainide (3 mg/kg), or propanolol (80 mg) plus diltiazem (120 mg).

VENTRICULAR TACHYCARDIAS
Diagnosis
Features are:

- Broad QRS
- Rate > 120 bpm
- Regular.

Be aware of other causes of broad complex tachycardias:

- Atrial fibrillation with irregular aberrant conduction
- Supraventricular tachycardia with aberrant conduction – this has capture or fusion beats (more common in exams!). The axis will be the same as the normal 12 lead.

Treatment
Emergency situation
If the patient is compromised (i.e. falling blood pressure, unwell, unconscious, no pulse) treat as a peri-arrest/arrest situation and follow the advanced life support algorithm.

Well patient in sustained ventricular tachycardia on the ward
Assuming the patient has a stable blood pressure and is well perfused:

- Move, if possible, to a monitored high-dependency unit bed
- Consider (and correct or remove) reversible causes:
  - Ischaemia (acute myocardial infarction)
  - Drugs (e.g. anti-arrhythmics)
  - Electrolyte imbalance (potassium, magnesium)
  - Thyroid dysfunction
  - Systemic upset (e.g. infection, malignancy).

Drugs
Consider:

- Amiodarone i.v. via a central or long line (300 mg over 1 hour, 900 mg over next 23 hours)
- Atenolol i.v. or lignocaine i.v. can also be used if this fails, but we would have a low threshold to try DC cardioversion at this point.

DC cardioversion

Perform as in the algorithm above. This is an emergency procedure so give a bolus of 5000 units of heparin i.v. followed by a
heparin infusion before cardioversion.

Implantable cardioverter defibrillator

Unless there was a clearly reversible cause, such as ischaemia, the
patient should receive an ICD.

Incidental pick-up on monitor or 24-hour tape

As above, look for reversible pathology by organising:

- An exercise-tolerance test (ischaemia)
- An echocardiogram (hypertrophic cardiomyopathy, dilated
  cardiomyopathy, certain congenital diagnoses, e.g. tetralogy of
  Fallot)
- Bloods.

Look for history of collapse or dizziness.

- A short run (e.g. < eight beats of asymptomatic ventricular
  tachycardia) in a patient with a normal heart does not need
  treatment. Beta blockers would be a wise precaution as would
  a follow-up 24-hour tape in 6–12 months
- Patients with longer or symptomatic runs of ventricular tachycardia should have an ICD, as should patients with impaired
  left ventricular function (see below).

IMPLANTABLE CARDIOVERTER DEFIBRILLATORS

Now little bigger than conventional pacemakers, ICDs are fitted in
the same way, usually under sedation rather than with formal
anaesthesia. Sedation is used (e.g. diamorphine and midazolam) to
allow the device to be tested. Ventricular fibrillation is induced via
the device and it is essential that the device then senses this and is
able to defibrillate the patient out of it easily within its energy
thresholds.

   If detecting ventricular fibrillation and ventricular tachycardias
is all that is needed, the device can use a right ventricular lead only

and will have algorithms to distinguish between supraventricular tachycardias and ventricular tachycardias. These are not infallible and in patients with frequent supraventricular tachycardias, most operators have a low threshold to place a right atrial lead to increase the device's diagnostic sensitivity.

The indications for ICD implantation have changed over the last 5 years as trial data become available, and it is necessary to understand a few trial data to see where we are now and to realise that we have not yet finished the journey. It is also worth remembering that sudden cardiac death is often the patient's first presentation, so primary prevention is far superior to secondary.

Trial data: primary prevention

The key studies are shown in **Table 30**. In the US, everyone who has had a myocardial infarction with an ejection fraction < 30% receives an ICD. MEDICARE states that these patients should not have had class IV heart failure or revascularisation in the last 3 months, or be about to undergo revascularisation. It is likely that we will follow in the UK.

In the DINAMIT study,[14] MADIT II type patients in a treatment group received an ICD early (< 40 days) after a myocardial infarction. Although arrhythmogenic deaths were reduced in the ICD

Table 30. Key trial data for ICDs: primary prevention	
MADIT[10]	Showed that patients who had had a myocardial infarction with an ejection fraction of < 35%, and inducible ventricular tachycardia benefited from an ICD
MUST[11]	Showed that electrophysiological studies were essentially a waste of time
MADIT II[12]	Patients with a previous myocardial infarction and an ejection fraction < 30% were the only inclusion criteria. The study showed patients benefited significantly with an ICD
SCD-HeFT[13]	Showed that in patients with MADIT II criteria, QRS duration did not discriminate high-risk patients

group, more deaths from non-arrhythmogenic causes occurred resulting in no significant differences between the two groups. Essentially, if you are very sick after a myocardial infarction, the ICD will prevent arrhythmia but not pump failure.

The conclusion is: don't rush straight in with your ICD. It would seem reasonable to allow at least a three-month delay before implantation.

Trial data: secondary prevention

The AVID, CIDS and CASH trials looked at patients who survived ventricular fibrillation or had symptomatic ventricular tachycardia.[15-17] They were less convincing than the primary prevention trials and needed a meta-analysis to achieve consistent significance. This was seen mostly in patients with an ejection fraction < 35%.

The European Society of Cardiology states that patients should receive an ICD in the following situations:

- If arrest was due to ventricular fibrillation or ventricular tachycardia and no obvious reversible cause
- Spontaneous sustained ventricular tachycardia in a structurally normal heart not amenable to other treatments
- Ventricular tachycardia with syncope or significant haemodynamic compromise
- Sustained ventricular tachycardia and an ejection fraction < 35%, but not worse than NYHA class III heart failure
- Hypertrophic cardiomyopathy and two risk factors, or ventricular tachycardia or fibrillation
- Arrhythmogenic right ventricular cardiomyopathy. Drugs are first-line treatment, but if there is collapse or if drug therapy fails to suppress arrhythmias, then an ICD is indicated
- Idiopathic dilated cardiomyopathy. The CAT trial indicated that even with an ejection fraction of 30% or less, the mortality from arrhythmias was low in this group, and ICDs should not be implanted unless patients have documented ventricular tachycardia[18]
- Patients with Brugada syndrome with a history of syncope, or evidence of ventricular tachycardia.

ADDITIONAL INFORMATION

Some points to remember are given in **Table 31**.

Recommendations for driving are as follows.

- Patients are allowed to drive if:
  - The device has been in situ for 6 months
  - The device has not delivered a shock
  - Any previous arrhythmias were not accompanied by incapacity
- Patients are not allowed to drive for 1 month after any revision has been made to the system
- Patients may drive 1 month after implantation if the ICD is for primary prevention
- Patients are not allowed to drive lorries, buses, heavy goods vehicles, etc.

MANAGING PATIENTS WITH AN ICD
The ICD patient with multiple shocks

The ICD prevents ventricular tachycardia by either:

- Anti-tachycardia pacing, where the ICD actively paces the ventricle at a high rate to 'capture', then reduces the rate to end the tachycardia, *or*
- Giving an internal shock.

Table 31. ICDs: points to remember

- An ICD is not a cure!
- Implantation is just the start of your problems, not the end
- Patients need 24-hour access to telephone helplines and the ability to interrogate the devices should they go off
- ICDs can inappropriately shock people and some patients may have significant psychological problems caused by the devices

If the ICD is giving multiple therapies, these may be appropriate (i.e. each shock is for ventricular tachycardia) or inappropriate (the ICD misinterprets the cardiac rhythm). A pacing interrogation by a pacing technician will help distinguish these.

The devices record and store endocardial ECGs of the incidents, but these cannot be read with the same clarity as epicardial traces, and sometimes make ventricular tachycardia and supraventricular tachycardia or bundle branch block difficult to distinguish.

Inappropriate shocks

These are usually due to fast atrial fibrillation. You should:

- Get the ICD checked by a technician to ensure the box and leads are working correctly
- Add sotalol/atenolol or amiodarone
- Increase digoxin or add the above drugs if the patient has permanent atrial fibrillation.

Most devices look at the rate rather than QRS duration. The ventricular tachycardia rate is often higher than the supraventricular tachycardia rate, and allows the treatment rate to be increased above the supraventricular tachycardia rate, while still being low enough to appropriately detect ventricular tachycardia.

Appropriate shocks

The ICD acts as a safety net to prevent sudden cardiac death from ventricular tachycardia or ventricular fibrillation. But it is always better not to have to use the net at all. Some patients will find their ICDs fire multiple times appropriately, sometimes as many as 100 times in a short period!

This can be a sign of a pre-morbid state, but often their ventricular tachycardia should be further treated with drugs. If these 'ventricular tachycardia storms' are weathered, the patient can usually continue to have a good quality of life.

Remember:
- Correct any electrolyte imbalance and other reversible causes (see above). Give magnesium anyway (unless the patient is known to already be at potentially toxic levels)
- Amiodarone and sotalol/atenolol are the anti-arrhythmic drugs of first choice. Reload if necessary
- Patients with heart failure should be on a beta blocker; ensure the dose is adequate. Carvedilol is a good choice. Titrate the dose up slowly to 25 mg bd.

If the patient is still getting ventricular tachycardias, you can use other anti-arrhythmics. These were given a bad press because of their conversely pro-arrhythmic activity in the CAST trial (in patients with ischaemic heart disease), but that was in patients without defibrillators.[19] Choices are:
- Lignocaine (by slow i.v. infusion if patient is still getting ventricular tachycardia)
- Propafenone
- Mexiletine (slow i.v. infusion if lignocaine is not tolerated; this can be converted to an oral dose).

Heart transplantation and ventricular assist devices

Emma Birks
Nick Fisher
John Pepper

INTRODUCTION

Remember, referrals made too late are always a tragedy. No-one will mind if your referral is too early (including the patient!) and this allows patients to be carefully monitored and serial data collected.

Many patients will need a transplant at a later date and serial data allow the optimal moment to be seized. The aim is to catch patients when they develop severe heart failure but before they develop secondary organ failure.

INDICATIONS FOR HEART TRANSPLANTATION

The main indications are:
- NYHA class III or IV heart failure
  - Common – ischaemic heart disease, cardiomyopathy
  - Rare – valvular heart disease
- Re-transplantation for chronic rejection
- Congenital heart disease.

ASSESSING PATIENTS FOR HEART TRANSPLANTATION

A 'to do' list is given in **Table 32**. Remember:
- It is important to fill out the heart transplant assessment protocol form produced by the transplant unit

Table 32. Assessment for heart transplantation

- 24-hour urinary collection for creatinine clearance and protein excretion
- Liver function tests
- Clotting
- Blood group
- Serology – hepatitis B and C, cytomegalovirus and HIV
- Exercise capacity (VO_2 max and VE/VCO_2 slope). The usual cut-off for acceptance on to the heart transplant waiting list is when the VO_2 max becomes ≤ 14 ml/kg/min
- Echocardiography
- Left and right heart catheterisation
- Toxoplasma and VDRL serology
- 24-hour tape recording for arrhythmias

- Patients who have had a previous blood transfusion or pregnancy may have pre-formed HLA antibodies that will react with donor antigens. You must send a sample of the patient's blood to the tissue typing department for testing against a panel of reactive antibodies
- The usual cut-off for acceptance to the heart transplant waiting list is when the VO_2 max becomes ≤ 14 ml/kg/min
- At the time of transplantation, echocardiographic ejection fraction is generally $\leq 20\%$.

RIGHT HEART CATHETERISATION

Right heart catheterisation is very important because both brain-death-related myocardial dysfunction in the donor and myocardial injury resulting from ischaemia during transportation of the donor heart, affect the right ventricle more than the left ventricle.

Therefore, donor hearts often show right ventricular failure in the early post-transplant period, particularly when transplanted into heart failure patients with a high pulmonary vascular resistance. Consequently during right heart catheterisation it is important to measure:

- Systolic and mean pulmonary artery pressure
- Wedge pressure – a reliable tracing is essential because many important decisions will result from this
- Pulmonary artery saturations and a Fick cardiac output – blood will need to be taken from the sidearm of the sheath for haemoglobin and arterial saturations
- Transpulmonary gradient (mean pulmonary artery pressure minus mean wedge pressure) – you can derive pulmonary vascular resistance from this (transpulmonary gradient/cardiac output).
- Arterial pressure.

Transpulmonary gradient

The transpulmonary gradient is generally a better indicator of right-sided pressures than pulmonary vascular resistance because the latter is influenced by the low cardiac output that many of these patients have. When the transpulmonary gradient is:

- < 12 mmHg the risk of developing right heart failure is low
- 12–14 mmHg the risk of developing right heart failure is borderline
- 14 mmHg reversibility testing using intravenous sodium nitroprusside should be performed. If the transpulmonary gradient falls with sodium nitroprusside the pulmonary hypertension is likely to be reversible and to respond to peri-operative nitric oxide.

Arterial pressure

This should also be recorded at catheterisation because the pulmonary artery systolic pressure, reflected as a proportion of systemic pressure, is also a useful clinical guide (e.g. when pulmonary artery systolic pressure is $\geq$ two-thirds systemic systolic blood pressure, pulmonary hypertension is severe).

The transpulmonary gradient and pulmonary artery pressures are also important when size-matching the donor heart to the recipient:

- If the transpulmonary gradient and pulmonary artery pressures are high, a heart from a larger-sized donor will be needed to cope with the high pulmonary artery pressures in the recipient
- If the transpulmonary gradient and pulmonary artery pressures are low, a similar-sized or slightly smaller donor can be used.

LEFT-HEART CATHETERISATION

Perform a coronary angiography, if this has not been done in the recent past, to confirm the underlying diagnosis and to make sure no further corrective coronary surgery is possible.

The donor organ shortage means that heart transplantation is now mainly limited to younger candidates with no secondary organ damage. A large proportion of heart failure is due to CHD, and these patients being assessed for transplantation can also be considered for alternative types of surgery (e.g. hibernation surgery with or without ventricular remodelling, passive restraint or correction of mitral regurgitation).

SURVIVAL AFTER HEART TRANSPLANTATION

Survival after heart transplantation is now around 80%, 70% and 50% at 1, 5 and 10 years, respectively. This has been improving worldwide over the last two decades. After the 20% mortality rate in the first year there is a constant rate of 4% per year. Unfortunately, the supply of donors has been decreasing and the current supply of organs from brain-dead donors does not meet the continually increasing demand of patients needing heart transplants.

Immunosuppression

In the first 3 days after a transplant, the patient is given a combination of:

- Antithymocyte globulin (ATG)
- Corticosteroids
- Azathioprine or mycophenolate.

Subsequently, patients are maintained on triple-therapy immuno-suppression consisting of:

· Ciclosporin/tacrolimus
· Mycophenolate/azathioprine
· Corticosteroids.

In about 90% of patients in our hospital corticosteroids are tapered and discontinued late after transplantation.

Factors that increase one-year mortality are:

· Age
· Ventilation before transplantation
· Donor age
· Long ischaemia time
· Female donor/male recipient
· Positive panel reactive antibodies
· Diagnosis other than ischaemic heart disease or cardiomyopathy.

Causes of mortality and other complications are given in **Table 33**.

Monitoring for acute rejection

This is done with:

· Electrocardiography
· Echocardiography
· Endomyocardial biopsies.

Rejection can cause impaired ventricular performance, low cardiac output and hypotension, which are often out of proportion to the grade of rejection and can result in significant morbidity and mortality.

Treating acute rejection

Treatment is as follows:

· Mild rejection – give i.v. methylprednisolone
· Severe rejection – give i.v. methylprednisolone plus ATG or monoclonal antibodies.

Table 33. Causes of mortality after heart transplantation

Causes of mortality in the first year:
- Primary graft failure (most common cause in the first 30 days after heart transplantation, being responsible for 30% of deaths during this period)
- Acute rejection
- Infection

Causes of mortality after the first year:
- CHD
- Malignancy

Other complications:
- Renal dysfunction
- Infection (see cytomegalovirus below)
- Hypertension
- Diabetes
- Malignancy (mostly skin tumours and lymphomas)

Note: Most complications following transplantation are related to the immunosuppressive therapy.

Cytomegalovirus

This is the most important cause of morbidity and mortality from infectious disease. Patients at high risk are those seronegative for cytomegalovirus (CMV) who receive a heart from a seropositive donor.

Treatment of clinical CMV is with a 10–14-day course of intravenous ganciclovir. This is effective in more than 90% of patients.

Transplant coronary disease

This is the major cause of death in patients surviving one year after transplantation and affects long-term function of the transplanted heart. It is an unusually accelerated form of coronary disease affecting both intramyocardial and epicardial coronary arteries. Pathological changes range from concentric fibrous intimal thickening to complicated atheromatous plaques. It is likely to be primarily an immune-mediated disease.

Although there is partial re-innervation of the cardiac allograft, most patients cannot experience typical angina pain associated with myocardial ischaemia and the first clinical manifestations are often ventricular arrhythmias, heart failure or sudden death. Therefore, repeated post-operative coronary angiography is performed for diagnostic and surveillance purposes.

Intravascular ultrasound is an alternative diagnostic tool because it monitors intimal thickening. Some patients with transplant coronary disease are suitable for angioplasty and a very few undergo revascularisation.

UNCONVENTIONAL HEART TRANSPLANTATION
Domino transplantation
Domino transplantation is a technique in which the heart from a recipient undergoing heart and lung transplantation for cystic fibrosis or pulmonary hypertension is transplanted into another recipient. This provides a heart with a conditioned right ventricle, which is advantageous to a recipient with a high transpulmonary gradient. It renders that recipient less likely to develop right-sided heart failure after transplantation and also contributes to the donor pool.

Heterotopic transplantation
This is when the recipient heart is not removed and the donor heart gives support to the failing left ventricle of the native heart. Heterotopic transplantation is performed when:
- There is an undersized donor
- The recipient has pulmonary hypertension
- It is felt that the native heart could contribute significantly to the circulation (especially after concomitant native heart surgery).

Contraindications to heterotopic transplantation include patients with:
- Significant dysrhythmias
- Prosthetic valves
- Left ventricular clot
- Severe angina
- Implantable defibrillators.

Specific complications that can occur after heterotopic heart transplantation are significant ventricular arrhythmias of the native heart and recurrent angina. Despite the lack of routine anticoagulation, thromboembolic events are uncommon.

After an initial improvement in all ventricular parameters, deterioration of the native heart after heterotopic transplantation is a problem. The recipient left ventricle ejects more effectively when it contracts out of phase with the donor left ventricle. However, this is rarely the situation because the two hearts beat independently of one another and the denervated donor heart tends to beat faster than the recipient. Therefore, to improve the function of the native heart, it can be useful to link the two hearts electrically to coordinate recipient heart systole during donor heart diastole.

CATHETERISATION DURING ASSESSMENT FOR LUNG TRANSPLANTATION

Remember:
- Right heart catheterisation is also important when deciding on single or double lung transplantation
- The pulmonary artery pressures and wedge pressure should be measured and the transpulmonary gradient calculated (mean pulmonary artery pressure minus mean wedge pressure)
- Measure Fick cardiac output and calculate pulmonary vascular resistance (transpulmonary gradient divided by cardiac output). If the pulmonary vascular resistance is high in the recipient, the hypertrophied recipient right ventricle will be used to pump against a high pressure, and if a normal donor lung is inserted pulmonary oedema may occur. Donor lungs tend to

be susceptible to pulmonary oedema following ischaemia-reperfusion injury and this worsens the effect. Therefore, if the patient has a high pulmonary vascular resistance they are more likely to need double lung transplantation, because with twice the lung volume pulmonary oedema does not seem to be a problem

- In patients older than 50 years coronary angiography should also be performed during an assessment for single and double lung transplantation to ensure there is no concomitant coronary disease
- If the patient is to undergo heart and lung transplantation, the pressures and coronary assessment are not important because both organs will be replaced. However, if considering the heart for use as a domino transplant (see above), an echocardiogram is important to assess the degree of pulmonary and tricuspid regurgitation, right ventricular hypertrophy and dilatation.

LEFT VENTRICULAR ASSIST DEVICES

If patients waiting for transplantation develop secondary organ failure they can either undergo implantation with a left ventricular assist device (LVAD), which will improve secondary organ function as a bridge to transplantation, or they may be deemed 'untransplantable' and maintained on medical therapy. The pressure of external audit to maintain a high one-year survival following transplantation affects case selection, which can be both a good thing, leading to a good outcome, and a bad thing in excluding high-risk groups that might otherwise have had a chance of survival.

Therefore, an increasing number of patients with heart failure need an LVAD for survival. These are usually patients with NYHA class IV heart failure, with deteriorating clinical status with evidence of secondary organ dysfunction in the context of low cardiac output despite appropriate medical treatment including inotropes and an intra-aortic balloon pump. Again, it is important to catch these patients early because once they have developed liver impairment (usually judged by a raised bilirubin) they will have clotting problems and their risk from the procedure is vastly increased.

The LVAD functions by helping the left ventricle without removal of the heart. The pumping mechanism relies on a pusher plate (HeartMate or Novocor) or impeller system (Jarvick, HeartMate II or DeBakey).

The HeartMate I is one of the most commonly used pumps because of its low thrombogenicity. It is an implantable, pulsatile LVAD, and owing to the unique lining and flow characteristics of this pump only minimal anticoagulation (with aspirin) is needed. Patients can be supported for extended periods with a relatively low risk of thrombo-embolism or mechanical failure.

The major early complications are bleeding and right heart failure. Infection is common and is the biggest impediment to long-term success. Device failure, thrombo-embolism and neurological dysfunction can also occur.

The Jarvick and DeBakey devices are smaller impeller pumps and surgical implantation is less traumatic, but they require anticoagulation with warfarin because they do not have a textured surface.

LVADs are generally used in patients with advanced heart failure as a bridge to transplantation. A number of these patients have shown significant improvement in myocardial function, which has been sufficient in some cases to allow explantation of the device. The exact proportion of these patients is still unknown. LVADs can also be permanently left in place as destination therapy, generally in patients with contraindications to transplantation.

Adult congenital heart disease

chapter 13

Susanna Price
Mike Mullen
Mike Gatzoulis

INTRODUCTION

ACHD comprises a growing population of adult patients with different and often complex cardiac diagnoses. They most often present with common cardiological problems, namely arrhythmias and heart failure. Investigation and management frequently differ from those of patients with structurally normal hearts, so don't dabble!

If you are in doubt about the correct diagnosis or management, seek expert advice from:

- The patients! They often know themselves better than you. Listen to them
- The on-call ACHD specialist registrar or consultant at the hospital that follows them up.

GENERAL ADMISSIONS

On admission, all patients should have:

- An ECG
- A chest X-ray (PA and lateral if RV-PA conduit or possibility of needing re-sternotomy)
- U&Es test (including magnesium)
- Glucose test
- Liver function tests
- Thyroid function tests
- Coagulation test (see below)
- 6-minute walk test (not if Eisenmenger/pulmonary hypertension with recent haemoptysis – discuss with senior colleagues).

They should also have:

- A transthoracic echocardiogram – when it is a new diagnosis, there is a recent change in symptoms or there is no recent echocardiogram available
- Haematinics – if cyanotic
- Blood cultures – if endocarditis is a possibility. Do not start antibiotics until positive cultures are available
- A pregnancy test – if the patient is a woman of childbearing age
- Serum and faecal alpha$_1$-antitrypsin – if the patient has a Fontan circulation and has ascites
- 24-hour creatinine clearance – for an admission for surgery where there is borderline cardiac output or if the patient is being considered for heart transplantation.

INRS FOR PATIENTS WITH HIGH HAEMOGLOBIN

Patients with high haemoglobin may get misleading, usually very high, INR results when the packed cell volume is > 65 l/l, due to relatively low plasma volumes resulting in a too high concentration of citrate. A citrate-adjusted sample (prepared by the haematology department once the packed cell volume is known) is required.

Note that blood must be taken using a needle and syringe because the Vacutainer system will not work once the vacuum has been broken to remove citrate from the sample.

IMAGING IN ACHD PATIENTS

Imaging patients with CHD is highly specialised. As with all imaging, the more information you give, the more informative the results are likely to be. You can obtain most information needed about anatomy and physiology from a transthoracic echocardiogram performed by an expert.

Occasionally, you may need additional information from a cardiac MRI. Note that patients with standard metallic valve prostheses can be scanned, but patients with pacemakers may not. See local guidelines for the main exclusions.

MAJOR INDICATIONS FOR ADMISSIONS
Cyanotic patients
These patients have Eisenmenger syndrome or pulmonary hypertension with right to left shunting via intra-cardiac communication. The main indication for admission is haemoptysis. This can be minor (more common) or major.

Minor haemoptysis
Remember:
- Always inform seniors of admission because minor haemoptysis may herald major haemoptysis
- Ensure i.v. access, administer high-flow O_2 and i.v. fluids, check bloods as above, especially coagulation (note need for citrate-adjusted sample) and emergency cross match
- If the patient has an antecedent history of chest infection, do blood cultures
- Specialist investigations include chest X-ray (compare with old films if available) and CT scanning (look for pulmonary artery thrombus and pulmonary haemorrhage)
- Management is usually conservative. Consider an antibiotic if the precipitant is infection. Stop warfarin temporarily. Advise bed/chair rest.

Major haemoptysis
Patients with massive haemoptysis usually die from failure to maintain their airway rather than massive blood loss. Major haemoptysis is a clinical emergency. Initial resuscitation must therefore involve a decision regarding intubation and ventilation, in addition to standard resuscitation for volume loss (i.v. volume, oxygen, bloods, etc as above) and involve seniors at the earliest opportunity.

Intravenous lines
Patients with right–left shunting are at significant risk from air embolisation when air enters the venous system. Take great care to avoid ingress of air when infusions are running, and use air filters.

Venesection

Many patients will have had venesection in the past. However, current evidence suggests that this may be detrimental. Patients may complain of symptoms due to relative iron deficiency (check haematinics), which will respond to oral or i.v. iron. Consider venesection only if patients have symptoms from erythrocytosis (headache, nosebleeds, sensation of congestion). Always ensure adequate volume replacement if venesection is undertaken.

Acyanotic patients

Effectively univentricular circulation

The most common indications for admission are arrhythmia and ventricular failure.

Arrhythmia

In the univentricular circulation, atrial and ventricular arrhythmias are poorly tolerated and should be regarded as an indication for urgent or emergency cardioversion. Macro-re-entrant atrial tachycardia is common and may be difficult to diagnose (especially if the atria are large) and comparison with previous ECGs or echocardiography may help make the correct diagnosis.

Investigations should include:
- ECG (compare with normal if available)
- Coagulation
- U&Es (potassium: 4.5–5.0 mmol/l, magnesium: 1.0 mmol/l)
- Chest X-ray
- Transthoracic echocardiography.

Look for precipitant factors (infection, non-compliance with anti-arrhythmic medication, alcohol, etc).

Management is as follows:
- Correct electrolyte disturbance
- Start heparin (if not adequately anticoagulated)
- DC cardioversion.

You will usually need transoesophageal echocardiography to exclude left-sided thrombus, but this is a senior decision. The patient may cardiovert to a more malignant rhythm or to asystole.

Note that some patients (e.g. those with a Fontan circulation) will have no venous access for ventricular pacing. You should therefore have external pacing available. The senior anaesthetist should sedate or anaesthetise the patient for the procedure.

Ventricular failure

Having a univentricular right ventricle is worse than having a univentricular left ventricle, but eventually all univentricular hearts will develop ventricular failure due to chronic volume overload. Investigations should exclude treatable causes (i.e. arrhythmia, conduit obstruction).

Management is as for any patient with heart failure, but these patients are often exquisitely sensitive to medication so you should introduce it cautiously while monitoring fluid balance, daily weights and renal function. Take care to avoid over-diuresis because this will result in circulatory collapse.

Fontan (and modified Fontan) circulation

This is a special consideration. In addition to the conditions above, most patients with a Fontan circulation will be anticoagulated because of the risk of developing thrombus in the giant right atrium.

Remember:
- If patients present with ascites, exclude obstruction of the Fontan circulation
- If the Fontan circulation is unobstructed, consider the diagnosis of protein-losing enteropathy.

Protein-losing enteropathy is diagnosed by measuring serum and faecal alpha$_1$-antitrypsin (ensure a faecal occult blood test is negative or abnormally high levels will be measured in the stool sample).

Discuss treatment with a senior clinician: consider steroids or UF heparin.

Biventricular circulation

The most common indications for admission are:

- Infective endocarditis
- Arrhythmias
- Ventricular failure.

Arrhythmias and ventricular failure should usually be treated as for patients with normal hearts. However, the benefit of ACE inhibitors in right ventricular failure is unproven.

Infective endocarditis

This may be difficult to diagnose and locate in patients with complex congenital heart disease.

- In patients with shunts (i.e. Blalock–Taussig) consider shunt endocarditis if no obvious infection can be seen in the heart.
- **ALWAYS** send blood cultures+++, and antibiotics should usually be withheld until the responsible organism is identified. **DO NOT** start antibiotics, therefore, without a positive culture unless on very senior advice.

Ensure the relevant congenital cardiac surgical team is aware of the admission. Endocarditis in this patient population is often a surgical disease.

Congenitally corrected transposition of the great arteries (double discordance)

This may present with systemic (right) ventricular failure, tachyarrhythmias or complete heart block (in patients in their 20s and 30s) with a slow ventricular escape rate. Complete heart block in this context is not usually an indication for emergency pacing. Senior operators only should perform permanent pacing where indicated.

Mustard/Senning

Consider baffle obstruction or baffle leaks. These are usually diagnosed with transthoracic echocardiography with or without cardiac catheterisation.

CARDIAC CATHETERISATION AND IMAGING

Erythrocytotic patients and those with effectively univentricular circulation are at increased risk of contrast media nephropathy, as well as circulatory collapse where fluids are withheld. Although measured urea and creatinine may be within the normal rage, the creatinine clearance is likely to be reduced. If in doubt it should be measured.

Any cyanosed patient or patients with an effectively univentricular circulation should have intravenous hydration before catheterisation, surgery or imaging necessitating 'nil by mouth'. The choice of fluid and rate of administration will be guided by the patient's electrolyte status, cardiac function and body mass index. Also consider pre-treatment with N-acetylcysteine.

PREGNANCY AND CONTRACEPTION

All women of childbearing age admitted should have a pregnancy test and be regarded as pregnant until proven otherwise.

The ideal management strategy for ACHD patients contemplating pregnancy is to have a pre-pregnancy assessment in a specialist joint clinic, with follow-up as appropriate throughout the pregnancy and the post-partum period.

Pregnancy is contraindicated in patients with Eisenmenger syndrome and with severe pulmonary hypertension. The next most high-risk patients are those with stenotic or obstructive lesions and patients with an effectively univentricular circulation. Marfan's syndrome presents a special problem because during pregnancy there may be sudden and unexpected aortic dilatation or dissection.

Because warfarin is potentially teratogenic, patients for whom anticoagulation is absolutely or strongly indicated should be admitted to hospital. Warfarin should be stopped and switched to either treatment doses of LMWH or UF heparin intravenously.

Many drugs are potentially teratogenic, but your primary duty of care is to the mother. Seek expert and senior advice about changing any medication in this situation, and document *everything*. You may be very glad that you did in a few years' time …

It is generally recommended that patients at risk of thrombosis avoid oestrogen-containing contraceptives. Alternatives include the progesterone-only pill and depot preparations. More modern intra-uterine devices are less likely to provoke menorrhagia, which is a concern in patients who are systemically anticoagulated. There is an additional theoretical risk of increasing the risk of endocarditis with an intra-uterine device in situ, especially when a patient is at high risk of endocarditis.

COMMON INTERVENTIONS
Device closure of secundum atrial septal defects

Device closure of secundum atrial septal defects (ASD) is now well established as a therapeutic tool. However, clinical follow-up remains short and the demographic characteristics of patients undergoing device closure are likely to differ from those of patients who traditionally would have been referred for surgery. Although most patients are young, a significant proportion are older and may already have established symptoms or concomitant cardiovascular disease.

Indications for device closure

Indications are:

- Secundum ASD ≤ 40 mm (stretched diameter) in the context of a left to right shunt (QP:QS > 1.5)
- Significant right heart volume load (right atrial and right ventricular dilatation)
- Paradoxical embolisation.

Contraindications are:

- ASD > 40 mm (stretched diameter)
- Insufficient inferior, superior or posterior rim (< 5 mm). Absence of aortic rim is acceptable
- Presence of ostium primum, sinus venosus or coronary sinus defect, or anomalous pulmonary venous drainage

- Other conditions that require cardiac surgery
- Presence of intracardiac thrombus, sepsis or decompensated heart failure
- Pulmonary hypertension with net right to left shunt and systemic desaturation.

Note that patients with pulmonary hypertension (pulmonary artery pressure > 75%) need reversibility studies. If there is a net left to right shunt they may still benefit from device closure, but careful follow-up is necessary.

Pre-procedure care
Document:
- Clinical and demographic data
- Age
- Sex
- History of dyspnoea, fatigue, arrhythmia or angina.

Carry out a physical examination.

Investigations should include:
- ECG – note rhythm, P wave and QRS axis, and QRS duration
- Chest X-ray
- Cardiothoracic ratio and pulmonary plethora
- MVO_2
- Echocardiography
- Cardiac catheterisation.

Echocardiography
In most patients a satisfactory assessment of ASD size, position and suitability for device closure and exclusion of other major abnormalities may be made by careful assessment with transthoracic echocardiography. Routine transoesophageal echocardiography is therefore not necessary before referral unless:

- Transthoracic echocardiography images are inadequate
- The defect is very large (> 3 cm)
- There is doubt about potential contraindications to device closure (i.e. partial anomalous pulmonary venous drainage).

A detailed assessment of the anatomy of the intra-atrial septum and associated structures will always be performed by transthoracic echocardiography or intracardiac ultrasound before attempting closure of the defect.

Cardiac catheterisation
Patients older than 40 years should have a pre-assessment of their coronary artery anatomy. A haemodynamic study should be performed to estimate left to right shunt and to measure pulmonary blood pressure.

Cardiac catheterisation should be performed in all patients with clinical or echocardiographic evidence of pulmonary hypertension. If pulmonary artery pressure is > 75% systemic, patients should have reversibility studies. Always consider other causes of pulmonary hypertension.

The risks of device closure are given in **Table 34**.

Table 34. Risks of device closure	
Death	< 1/500
Stroke	1/100 (atrial fibrillation) 1/500 (sinus rhythm)
Device embolisation	< 1/100
Arrhythmia	1/50
Transient chest pain and ST elevation	< 1/100
Headache or migraine	1/30

Peri-procedure care

Device closure is performed using fluoroscopic and echocardiographic guidance. A general anaesthetic is needed if using transoesophageal echocardiography. A local anaesthetic is sufficient if intracardiac ultrasound is used.

Before the procedure carry out a brief clinical history and examination. All patients should have an ECG.

Drugs
- All patients should start an antiplatelet regime 24 hours before the procedure
  - Aspirin 150 mg/day for 6 months
  - Clopidogrel 150 mg loading followed by 75 mg/day for 6 weeks
- Stop warfarin 4 days before the procedure and restart immediately afterwards
- Clopidogrel can be omitted in patients on warfarin
- Patients in atrial fibrillation should be heparinised for 24 hours after device deployment while warfarin is restarted.

Post-procedure care

Remember:
- Provide normal groin care
- Once ambulant perform a chest X-ray (PA & Lat) and ECG. Record device position and rhythm
- Perform an echocardiogram to confirm satisfactory device deployment and exclude pericardial effusion
- Some patients may be suitable for discharge on the same day.

Follow-up

At 6 weeks order:
- An ECG
- A chest X-ray
- An echocardiogram to confirm device position and presence or absence of residual leaks.

Record the presence or absence of complications.

At 1 and 3 years order:
- An ECG
- A chest X-ray
- Detailed transthoracic echocardiography
- MVO_2.

Stenting of coarctation of the aorta

Intravascular stents have recently been employed as a non-surgical approach to treating aortic coarctation. Although the haemodynamic results are favourable, the overall effect on arterial and cardiac structure and function has not been assessed.

Indications

There are no rigid indications for intervention in patients with native or re-coarctation. Factors taken into account include:

- Anatomy – optimal results are achieved with discrete coarctation/re-coarctation distal to the left subclavian. In this situation stenting may be the treatment of choice. However, satisfactory results may also be achieved in patients with near interruption, and those with hypoplastic arches or isthmus or long-segment stenosis. Consider each case on its own merits
- Upper body hypertension (may be present despite adequate relief of coarctation)
- Pressure gradient > 15 mmHg (a low gradient may be present if there are good collaterals; however, this may not imply a satisfactory haemodynamic condition)
- Diastolic flow on Doppler or MRI (may be reduced if proximal aorta is stiff)
- Aortic regurgitation
- Left ventricular hypertrophy
- CHD.

There are no absolute contraindications. Take care when considering patients with a previous Dacron patch repair.

Pre-procedure care

Document:

- Clinical and demographic data
- Age
- Sex
- History of dyspnoea, fatigue, arrhythmia, angina.

Carry out a physical examination and record blood pressure in both arms and in the lower body.

Investigations are as follows:

- Fasting blood for lipids and glucose
- ECG
- Chest X-ray
- Exercise test (blood pressure monitoring)
- 24-hour blood pressure monitor
- Transthoracic echocardiography (to confirm the diagnosis and exclude other pathology, and to assess left ventricular function, dimensions and mass, and severity of aortic regurgitation)
- MRI (to assess anatomy, left ventricular function and mass, severity of aortic regurgitation, aortic compliance and distensibility).

The risks of stenting of coarctation are given in **Table 35**.

Table 35. Risks of stenting of coarctation	
Mild transient non-specific chest pain	Very common
Aortic dissection/rupture	1/100
Death	1/100
Stroke	1/200
Stent malposition	< 1/30
Vascular complication requiring intervention	1/100
Aneurysm formation*	1/20
*This may not be clinically apparent until follow-up	

Peri-procedure care

Remember:

- Coarctation stenting is performed with the patient under general anaesthesia using fluoroscopic guidance
- Perform a brief clinical history and examination before the procedure
- All patients should have an ECG before the procedure
- Stop warfarin 4 days before the procedure
- Routine clerking and bloods should be performed. *All patients MUST have blood sent for cross match.*

Post-procedure care

Remember:

- Provide normal groin care (let cardiologists know if pulses are absent)
- Monitor blood pressure
- Many patients experience a mild non-specific chest pain
- Once the patient is ambulant perform a chest X-ray (PA & Lat) and ECG. Record stent position; note presence of mediastinal widening or new pleural effusion
- Most patients will be suitable for discharge the next day
- Continue antihypertensive medication
- Organise contrast-enhanced spiral CT for follow-up.

Follow-up

At six weeks:

- Order an ECG
- Order a chest X-ray
- Review spiral CT
- Order an echocardiogram to confirm stent position and gradient
- Record presence or absence of complications
- Consider need for ongoing antihypertensive medication.

At 9–12 months order:
- An ECG
- A chest X-ray
- An echocardiogram
- A 24-hour blood pressure assessment
- An exercise test with blood pressure monitoring
- An MRI (as above)
- Cardiac catheterisation.

At 2 years order:
- An ECG
- A chest X-ray
- An echocardiogram
- A 24-hour blood pressure assessment.

Further imaging with MRI or spiral CT is appropriate in patients who have evidence of aneurysm formation.

Important and common drug interactions

Bilal Iqbal
Janet Lock
Nick Fisher

INTRODUCTION

Cardiology patients frequently have extensive medication lists. Statistically, if you take six different drugs there is an 80% chance of at least one drug interaction. It is no good congratulating yourself for curing paroxysmal atrial fibrillation with amiodarone and then finding that the patient died of a haemorrhage with an INR of 10!

You should be intimately aware of the interactions of warfarin, digoxin, amiodarone and statins. We have therefore discussed these in some detail and have provided a reference table for everyday use.

WARFARIN

Whenever you start warfarin or give a new drug to a patient taking warfarin, you must be aware which drugs increase or decrease its effect. Drugs that increase the effect of warfarin are given in **Table 36.**

Drugs that decrease the effect of warfarin include:
- Phenytoin (can send INR up or down so watch out)
- Carbamazepine
- Barbiturates
- Rifampicin
- Theophyllines
- Sulphonylureas (glibenclamide and tolbutamide).

Table 36. Drugs that increase the effects of warfarin

Drug	Mechanism of interaction	Comments
Amiodarone	Inhibits warfarin metabolism and displaces warfarin from binding sites	A 30–50% reduction in warfarin may be needed. The enhanced anticoagulant effect may be delayed, requiring close monitoring for 2–4 weeks. Due to the long half-life of amiodarone, the effect may persist for months following discontinuation of warfarin
Simvastatin	Inhibits warfarin metabolism	Decrease doses of warfarin by 30%. Atorvastatin and pravastatin do not appear to interact with warfarin
Aspirin	Increased risk of bleeding due to anti-platelet action and gastric erosions	Depending on clinical scenario, aspirin may be discontinued on initiation of warfarin therapy
Clopidogrel	Increased risk of bleeding due to anti-platelet action and gastric erosions	Do not withdraw from patients after stent implantation unless cardiologist informed
NSAIDs	Increased risk of bleeding due to anti-platelet action and gastric erosions	Try to avoid. For analgesic effects consider paracetamol or codydramol
Fenofibrate	Mechanism not established	INR can increase
Erythromycin, clarithromycin and azithromycin	Inhibits warfarin metabolism, and the action of warfarin may be prolonged due to alterations in intestinal flora and its production of vitamin K for clotting factor production	This interaction is highly probable, but is often delayed for several days. The interaction is less with azithromycin
Ciprofloxacin, ofloxacin and levofloxacin	Action of warfarin may be prolonged due to alterations in intestinal flora and its production of vitamin K for clotting factor production	Monitor INR and adjust warfarin dose as necessary
Metronidazole	Inhibits warfarin metabolism	Monitor INR and reduce warfarin dose as necessary, which is usually by 30%
Fluconazole and itraconazole	Inhibits warfarin metabolism	Monitor INR and adjust warfarin dose as necessary
Allopurinol	Unknown	INR can shoot up in a few individuals
Tamoxifen	Unknown	Monitor INR and reduce warfarin dose as necessary, which is usually by 30%

STATINS

The main concern is myopathy (myositis and rhabdomyolysis), especially at high plasma levels.

Don't get these three confused:
- Myalgia – muscle aches and weakness *without* elevated creatinine kinase
- Myositis – muscle symptoms *with* elevated creatinine kinase
- Rhabdomyolysis – muscle symptoms *with* elevated creatinine kinase (> 10 x ULN), usually with raised creatinine, and myoglobinuria.

Risk factors

Risk factors for myopathy are:
- Renal impairment
- Untreated hypothyroidism
- Alcohol abuse
- Age > 70 years
- Underlying muscle disorders
- Chinese or Japanese descent
- Previous history of myopathy with statins/fibrates
- Concurrent use of fibrates, niacin or ciclosporin.

Remember:
- Serum transaminase concentrations can transiently rise and statins should be stopped if they remain persistently higher than three times reference values
- Myopathy is a rare but significant complication. Statins should be discontinued if creatinine kinase is five times higher than normal levels
- Simvastatin potentiates the effect of warfarin; often a 30% decrease in the warfarin dose is needed.

Contraindications

Important contraindications are:

- Active liver disease (transaminases > 3 x ULN)
- Pregnancy and breast feeding
- Women of childbearing age, unless it is highly unlikely that they will become pregnant.

Drugs that increase simvastatin levels are given in **Table 37**.

DIGOXIN

Digoxin is commonly prescribed for patients, and the incidence of digoxin toxicity is 7–20%. Risk factors for digoxin toxicity include:

- Hypokalaemia
- Hypomagnesaemia
- Hypercalcaemia
- Hypothyroidism
- Concurrent drug therapy (see below).

Table 37. Drugs that increase simvastatin levels*	
Drug	**Recommendation**
Azole antifungals, macrolides, HIV protease inhibitors	• Avoid simvastatin • Exercise caution with atorvastatin • Stop statin during therapy and for 2 days post-therapy
Ciclosporin, fibrates	• Do not exceed simvastatin 10 mg • Exercise caution with atorvastatin
Verapamil, amiodarone	• Do not exceed simvastatin 20 mg • Exercise caution with atorvastatin
Diltiazem	• Do not exceed simvastatin 40 mg
Grapefruit juice	• Avoid simvastatin • Avoid > 200 ml with atorvastatin
(*and atorvastatin to a lesser extent)	

Digoxin levels

Maintain therapeutic digoxin levels between 0.8 and 2.5 nmol/l (1–2 ng/ml). Samples for digoxin levels should be taken 6 hours after the last dose. Levels > 2.5 nmol/l are associated with digoxin toxicity.

Digoxin toxicity

Symptoms include:
- Gastrointestinal symptoms (nausea and vomiting, anorexia, abdominal pain and diarrhoea)
- Muscle weakness
- Fatigue
- Disorientation
- Visual disturbances (blurred vision, photophobia, dilated pupils and yellow vision)
- Tachy- and bradyarrhythmias.

ECG changes include:
- T-wave inversion
- ST depression
- Increased PR interval
- Ectopics
- Nodal rhythm
- Atrial fibrillation
- Ventricular tachycardia.

Managing digoxin toxicity

Management is as follows:
- Stop digoxin
- Send an urgent sample for digoxin, potassium, magnesium and calcium levels
- Correct electrolyte disturbances
- Correct arrhythmia
- For massive digoxin overdose or refractory digitalis toxicity, use Digibind (stored at regional centres)
  - 40 mg/vial; calculate vials needed based on digoxin level
  - Vials = [digoxin level in ng/ml] x [weight (kg)/100].

Drugs that increase digoxin levels are given in **Table 38.**

Table 38. Drugs that increase digoxin levels		
Drug	**Mechanism of interaction**	**Comments**
Amiodarone	Displaces digoxin from binding sites and decreases the clearance of digoxin	Obtain digoxin level before starting amiodarone. Then decrease digoxin dose by 50%. Monitor digoxin levels weekly for several weeks
Thiazide and loop diuretics	Increase risk of digoxin toxicity by hypokalaemia and/or hypomagnesaemia	Monitor electrolytes and correct as necessary
Erythromycin and clarithromycin	Increase digoxin levels by altering gastrointestinal flora, which leads to increased absorption of digoxin	Toxicity not common, but be aware of its possibility
Verapamil and diltiazem	Decrease tubular clearance of digoxin	Monitor digoxin levels. Need to reduce dose by 50% if verapamil dose is $\geq$ 160 mg
Spironolactone	Unknown	Increases digoxin levels by 25%

AMIODARONE

Amiodarone has several electrophysiological effects. These can manifest on the ECG as:

- Sinus bradycardia
- Increased PR interval
- Increased QRS duration
- Increased QT interval.

Adverse reactions due to amiodarone are not uncommon. Because of its long half-life (around 100 days) amiodarone toxicity is difficult to manage, compared with toxicity from drugs with shorter half-lives. Adverse effects can be divided into early and late. Early toxicity commonly occurs during the early loading dose phases of amiodarone.

Early toxicity
Effects include:
- Gastrointestinal upset (anorexia, nausea and vomiting)
- Sinus bradycardia and heart block
- Constitutional symptoms (malaise and fatigue)
- Neurological symptoms (dizziness and ataxia).

Late toxicity
Effects include:
- Pulmonary fibrosis (can occur from 2 weeks to 3 years after starting therapy)
- Skin (ultraviolet light hypersensitivity and slate-grey skin discoloration)
- Thyroid dysfunction (hypo- and hyperthyroidism)
- Corneal microdeposits
- Hepatotoxicity (rarely, hepatic necrosis and failure).

Drugs that interact with amiodarone are given in **Table 39**.

OTHER IMPORTANT DRUG INTERACTIONS
In a drug interaction, the *precipitant drug* causes an altered effect in the *object drug*. **Table 40** lists other common drug interactions encountered in cardiology patients. A quick reference to drug interactions is given in **Table 41**.

Table 39. Drugs that interact with amiodarone

Drug	Mechanism of interaction	Comment
Warfarin	Decreased metabolism and displacement from binding sites, causing an increased anticoagulant effect	Monitor INR. A 25–30% dose reduction in warfarin is recommended
Digoxin	Potentiates digoxin toxicity. Synergistic depression of the sino-atrial node and AV node, causing bradycardia and heart block	Monitor heart rate and blood pressure. A 50% dose reduction in digoxin is recommended
Beta blockers	Bradycardia and heart block	Monitor heart rate and blood pressure. A 50% dose reduction in beta blocker is recommended. Would not use sotalol
Verapamil	Bradycardia and heart block	Monitor heart rate and blood pressure. A 30% dose reduction in verapamil is recommended
Ciclosporin	Inhibition of ciclosporin metabolism leading to increased ciclosporin levels, potentiating ciclosporin toxicity	Monitor ciclosporin levels. Maximum dose 10 mg
Flecainide	Unknown	Reduce dose by 50%
Simvastatin	Reduced simvastatin metabolism	Reduce dose to 20 mg maximum
Phenytoin	Reduced phenytoin metabolism	Reduce dose if blood levels indicate

Table 40. Other important drug interactions

Precipitant drug	Object drug	Mechanism of interaction	Comment
ACE inhibitors	Lithium	Elevated lithium levels	Monitor lithium levels
NSAIDs	ACE inhibitors	NSAIDs may reduce hypotensive effect	Monitor blood pressure and renal function
Verapamil	Ciclosporin	Decreased ciclosporin metabolism leading to increased levels	Monitor ciclosporin levels
Thiazide diuretics	Lithium	Decreased renal clearance leading to increased lithium levels	Monitor lithium levels

Table 41. Reference guide to drug interactions

	Warfarin	Amiodarone	Digoxin	Statin	Beta blocker	Diltiazem
Warfarin		↑ INR		↑ INR		
Amiodarone	↑INR		↑ digoxin	↑ statin*	↓ HR, AV block	↓ HR, AV block
Digoxin		↑ digoxin			↓ HR, AV block	
Statin	↑ INR	↑ statin*				↑ statin*
Beta blocker		↓ HR, AV block	↓ HR, AV block			↓ HR, AV block
Diltiazem		↓ HR, AV block		↑ statin*	↓ HR, AV block	
Verapamil		↓ HR, AV block	↑ digoxin	↑ statin*	↓ HR, AV block, ↓ BP	↓ HR, AV block, ↓ BP
Propafenone			↑ digoxin		↑beta blocker	
Quinidine		↑ quinidine	↑ digoxin		↑beta blocker	

AV = atrioventricular; BP = blood pressure; HR = heart rate; INR = international normalised rat

Verapamil	Propafenone	Quinidine	Cimetidine**	Macrolides
			↑ INR	↑ INR
↓ HR, AV block		↑ quinidine		
↑ digoxin	↑ digoxin			↑ digoxin
↑ statin*				↑ statin* (AVOID)
↓ HR, AV block, ↓ BP	↑ beta blocker	↑ beta blocker	↑ beta blocker	
↓ HR, AV block, ↓ BP				
		↑ quinidine		
		↑ propafenone	↑ propafenone	
↑ quinidine	↑ propafenone		↑ quinidine	

*Only affects simvastatin and atorvastatin

**Such interactions have not been reported with ranitidine and proton pump inhibitors

Pre-operative cardiac evaluation for non-cardiac surgery

chapter 15

Bilal Iqbal
Nick Fisher

INTRODUCTION

The main purpose of assessing the cardiac status of a patient before non-cardiac surgery is to decide whether they need further cardiac assessment or intervention, before proceeding to surgery.

The preliminary assessment should include:
- Patient history
- Assessment of functional status
- Urgency of surgery
- Nature of the proposed surgery
- 12-lead ECG.

This will determine:
- Peri-operative cardiovascular risk
- Surgery-specific risk
- Patient's functional capacity.

You can use these three factors to decide which patients will benefit from further cardiac assessment and intervention by using the algorithm for pre-operative cardiac evaluation at the end of the chapter.

Peri-operative cardiovascular risk

This is based on patient's history, ECG, co-morbidities and clinical factors. It aims to stratify patients into major, intermediate or low risk for surgery.

Major risk

This is indicated by the following:

- Unstable coronary syndromes
  - Acute myocardial infarction (within the last 7 days)
  - Recent myocardial infarction (within the last month)
  - Unstable or severe angina (NYHA class III or IV heart failure)
- Decompensated heart failure
- Significant arrhythmias
  - High-grade AV block
  - Symptomatic ventricular arrhythmias with underlying heart disease
  - Supraventricular arrhythmias with uncontrolled ventricular rates
- Severe valvular heart disease.

Intermediate risk

This is indicated by the following:

- Mild angina pectoris
- Previous history of myocardial infarction
- Presence of pathological Q waves on an ECG
- Compensated or prior heart failure
- Diabetes mellitus (especially insulin-dependent)
- Renal insufficiency.

Low risk

This is indicated by the following:

- Advanced age
- ECG abnormalities (left ventricular hypertrophy, left bundle branch block or ST-T abnormalities)

- Rhythms other than sinus (e.g. atrial fibrillation/flutter)
- Low functional capacity (see below)
- History of stroke
- Uncontrolled systemic hypertension.

Surgery-specific risk

This is the risk associated with the type of surgery itself, irrespective of patient factors.

It can be classified into high-, intermediate- or low-risk surgery.

High-risk surgery (cardiac risk $\geq$ 5%)

This is indicated by the following:
- Major emergency surgery (especially in the elderly)
- Aortic or major vascular surgery
- Peripheral vascular surgery
- Procedures with large fluid shifts and/or blood loss.

Intermediate-risk surgery (cardiac risk 1–5%)

This is indicated by the following:
- Intraperitoneal and intrathoracic surgery
- Carotid endarterectomy
- Head and neck surgery
- Orthopaedic surgery
- Prostate surgery.

Low-risk surgery (cardiac risk < 1%)

This is indicated by the following:
- Endoscopic procedures
- Superficial biopsy
- Cataract surgery
- Breast surgery.

Patient's functional capacity

This is based on the patient's history and a direct assessment of functional status. The history should assess the patient's functional status, i.e. their ability to climb the stairs, to manage basic house-work and to perform regular exercise. Functional capacity can be expressed in metabolic equivalent (MET) levels. Energy expenditures for different activities correspond to different MET levels (**Table 42**).

Patients who are unable to meet a demand of 4 METs during normal daily activities are associated with increased peri-operative cardiac risk. Patients who are able to exercise on a regular basis without limitations generally have sufficient cardiovascular reserve to withstand surgery.

FURTHER CARDIAC ASSESSMENT

When deciding which patients are most likely to benefit from pre-operative cardiac assessment and treatment, consider the following points.

- Pre-operative testing should be limited to circumstances in which the results will affect the patient's treatment and outcome.
- Patients who have low-risk clinical predictors, good functional status and are undergoing low-risk surgery generally do not need further evaluation.
- Patients with high-risk clinical predictors and poor functional status who are being considered for high-risk surgery are more likely to benefit from further evaluation.

Table 42. Metabolic equivalent levels	
METs	**Activity**
1–4	Eating, dressing, walking around the house
4–10	Climbing stairs, walking up a hill, walking on level ground at 4 mph, running a short distance, playing a game of golf
> 10	Swimming, playing tennis, playing football, skiing

Pre-operative coronary angioplasty

Elective coronary revascularisation in low-risk patients who have stable coronary artery disease does not provide a survival benefit and does not reduce the risk of late myocardial infarction, compared with medical and preventative therapies.

Pre- and peri-operative beta blockers

Peri-operative stress is associated with sympathetic activation, which may provoke cardiac complications. By interrupting this cascade, peri-operative beta blockade has beneficial effects on cardiac function.

Beta blockade is associated with a significant reduction in the incidence of peri-operative myocardial ischaemia. You should titrate the dose to achieve a target heart rate of 60 bpm.

The indications for peri-operative beta blockers (given that there are no contraindications) are as follows:

- Patients undergoing high-risk surgery
- Ischaemic heart disease
- Heart failure
- Diabetes mellitus (especially insulin-dependent).

Hypertension

Systolic blood pressures $\geq$ 180 mmHg and diastolic blood pressures $\geq$ 110 mmHg should be controlled before surgery. You should establish an effective antihypertensive regimen in the weeks before surgery as an outpatient (see Chapter 6).

Valvular heart disease

Symptomatic aortic and mitral stenosis is associated with a high peri-operative risk. Discuss percutaneous valvotomy or valve replacement before non-cardiac surgery to lower cardiac risk.

Risk is greatest with aortic stenosis, where haemodynamic derangements during surgery that lower the blood pressure can cause a cardiac arrest. Significant aortic stenosis can make resuscitation extremely difficult.

Symptomatic valvular regurgitation is better tolerated and may be stabilised pre-operatively with intensive medical therapy and monitoring. Peri-operative hypertension is associated with increased valvular regurgitation that may result in congestive heart failure. Therefore, it is important to give effective peri-operative vasodilator therapy to reduce the afterload.

Discuss valve replacement before non-cardiac surgery in patients with reduced left ventricular function.

Arrhythmias

Start therapy for symptomatic or haemodynamically significant arrhythmias. Indications for therapy are similar to those in non-operative settings (see Chapter 11). Patients with atrial fibrillation/flutter have no contraindications to surgery if they are adequately rate-controlled. Frequent ventricular ectopics or asymptomatic non-sustained VT is not associated with an increased cardiac risk in the peri-operative period.

Conduction abnormalities

Patients with intra-ventricular conduction defects and bifascicular block, with or without first-degree AV block, should not have temporary pacing if there are no symptoms of syncope or documented episodes of advanced AV block.

The indications for temporary pacing are similar to those for permanent pacing, namely advanced AV block and severe symptomatic bradycardia. Such patients should have permanent pacemakers inserted before surgery.

An algorithm for determining which patients will benefit from invasive or non-invasive cardiac evaluation is given in **Figure 5**.

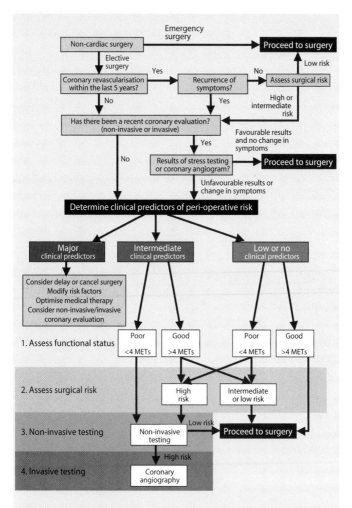

NB: Patients with a history of heart failure, known or suspected valvular heart disease or dyspnoea of unknown origin should have an echocardiogram.

Figure 5. Algorithm for deciding which patients will benefit from invasive/non-invasive coronary evaluation. Adapted from *J Am Coll Cardiol* 2002;39:542–53 with permission from the American College of Cardiology Foundation.

Appendix 1: Keeping up to date

Remember, in today's world of internet access there is no excuse for not to being up to date in your specialty.

- All the leading cardiology journals will, via their websites, email you the table of contents for their journals each month for free.
- It is most likely that your hospital or university will have internet access to these journals through their libraries and will provide you with the appropriate passwords to gain full text articles.
- **www.amedeo.com** is a very good website that you can configure to email you listings of articles published in journals of your choice and relevant to your specialty or subspecialty.
- These websites also email topical articles and contain much useful information:
  www.medscape.com
  www.theheart.org
  www.cardiosource.com

Finally, don't forget the major cardiology websites, which I've listed below.

American Heart Association	**www.americanheart.org**
Blood Pressure Association	**www.bpassoc.org.uk**
British Cardiac Society	**www.bcs.com**
British Hypertension Society	**www.bhsoc.org**

Cardiomyopathy Association	www.cardiomyopathy.org
European Heart Network	www.ehnheart.org
European Society of Cardiology	www.escardio.org
Global Cardiology Network	www.globalcardiology.org
Heart and Stroke Foundation of Canada	www.heartandstroke.ca
Hearts For Life	www.heartsforlife.co.uk
Mended Hearts (USA)	www.mendedhearts.org
National Heart Forum	www.heartforum.org.uk
National Heart Foundation of Australia	www.heartfoundation.com.au
National Heart, Lung, and Blood Institute (USA)	www.nhlbi.nih.gov
Pulmonary Hypertension Association (USA)	www.phassociation.org
Resuscitation Council (UK)	www.resus.org.uk
World Heart Day	www.worldheartday.com
World Heart Federation	www.worldheart.org

1. Malmberg K, Ryden L, Hamsten A *et al*. Randomized trial of insulin-glucose infusion followed by subcutaneous insulin treatment in diabetic patients with acute myocardial infarction (DIGAMI study): effects on mortality at 1 year. *J Am Coll Cardiol* 1995:26:56–65

2. European Society of Hypertension–European Society of Cardiology Guidelines Committee. 2003 European Society of Hypertension–European Society of Cardiology guidelines for the management of arterial hypertension. *J Hypertens* 2003;21:1011–1053. Also available at: www.escardio.org

3. National Institutes of Health. Seventh Report of the Joint National Committee on Prevention, Detection, Evaluation, and Treatment of High Blood Pressure (JNC 7). Bethesda, MD: NIH, August 2004. Also available at: www.nhlbi.nih.gov/guidelines/hypertension

4. Williams B, Poulter NR, Brown MJ *et al*. BHS guidelines working party, for the British Hypertension Society. British Hypertension Society guidelines for hypertension management 2004 (BHS-IV): summary. *BMJ* 2004;328:634–640. Also available at: www.bhsoc.org

5. ALLHAT Collaborative Research Group. Major outcomes in high risk, hypertensive, patients randomised to angiotensin converting enzyme inhibitor or calcium channel blocker versus diuretic. *J Am Med Assoc* 2002;288:2981–2997. Also available at: http://allhat.sph.uth.tmc.edu

6. Sever PS, Dahlof B, Poulter NR *et al*. The Anglo-Scandinavian cardiac outcomes trial: morbidity-mortality outcomes in the blood pressure lowering arm of the trial (ASCOT–BPLA). American College of Cardiology Annual Scientific Session 2005, March 6–9, Orlando, Florida. Late Breaking Clinical Trials

7. Department of Health. National service framework for coronary heart disease. London: DoH, 2000. Also available at: www.dh.gov.uk

8. Gregoratos G, Cheitlin MD, Conill A *et al*. ACC/AHA guidelines for implantation of cardiac pacemakers and antiarrhythmia devices. A report of the American College of Cardiology/American Heart Association Task Force on Practice Guidelines (Committee on Pacemaker Implantation). *Circulation* 1998;97:1325–1335. Also available at: www.americanheart.org

9. Blomstrom-Lundqvist C, Scheinman MM, Aliot EM *et al*. ACC/AHA/ESC guidelines for the management of patients with supraventricular arrhythmias. A report of the American College of Cardiology/American Heart Association Task Force and the European Society of Cardiology Committee for Practice Guidelines. Bethesda, MD: American College of Cardiology Foundation, 2003. Also available at: www.acc.org

10. Moss AJ, Hall WJ, Cannom DS *et al*. Improved survival with an implanted defibrillator in patients with coronary disease at high risk for ventricular arrhythmia. *N Engl J Med* 1996;335:1933–1940

11. Buxton A, Hafley G, Lee K *et al*. Relation of ejection fraction and inducible ventricular tachycardia to mode of death in patients with coronary artery disease: an analysis of patients enrolled in the Multicenter Unsustained Tachycardia trial. *Circulation* 2002;106:2466–2472

12. Moss AJ, Zarebra W, Hall WJ *et al*. Prophylactic implantation of a defibrillator in patients with myocardial infarction and reduced ejection fraction. *N Engl J Med* 2002;346:877–883

13. Bardy GH, Lee KL, Mark DB *et al*. Amiodarone or an implantable cardioverter-defibrillator for congestive heart failure. *N Engl J Med* 2005;352:225–237

14. Hohnloser SH, Kuck KH, Dorian P *et al* for the DINAMIT Investigators. Prophylactic use of an implantable cardioverter-defibrillator after acute myocardial infarction. *N Engl J Med* 2004;351:2481–2488

15. The Antiarrhythmics Versus Implantable Defibrillators (AVID) Investigators. A comparison of antiarrhythmic-drug therapy with implantable defibrillators in patients resuscitated from near-fatal ventricular arrhythmias. *N Engl J Med* 1997;337:1576–1583

16. Connolly SJ, Gent M, Roberts RS *et al.* Canadian Implantable Defibrillator Study (CIDS): a randomized trial of the implantable cardioverter defibrillator against amiodarone. *Circulation* 2000;101:1297–1302

17. Kuck KH, Cappato R, Siebels J *et al.* Randomized comparison of antiarrhythmic drug therapy with implantable defibrillators in patients resuscitated from cardiac arrest: the Cardiac Arrest Study Hamburg (CASH). *Circulation* 2000;102:748–754

18. Bänsch D, Antz M, Boczor S *et al.* Primary prevention of sudden death in idiopathic dilated cardiomyopathy: the Cardiomyopathy Trial (CAT). *Circulation* 2002;105:1453–1458

19. Echt DS, Liebson PR, Mitchell LB *et al.* Mortality and morbidity in patients receiving encainide, flecainide, or placebo: the Cardiac Arrhythmia Suppression Trial. *N Engl J Med* 1991;324:781–788

Index